Are the Blueberries in Your Waffles Really Blueberries?

A One-of-a Kind Guide to Eating Smart

Celeste C. Bumpus

Are the Blueberries in Your Waffles Really Blueberries?

Celeste C. Bumpus

Copyright © 2008 by
Celeste C. Bumpus

All rights reserved. No part of this book may be reproduced in any form by any means without permission in writing from the author.

Creative Publishing, Limited Company
21001 N. Tatum Blvd, Ste. 1630-458
Phoenix, Arizona 85050

Book Design by Peri Poloni-Gabriel,
Knockout Design, www.knockoutbooks.com

Editing by Patricia Brosio Adamson

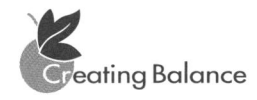

Creating Balance

Seminars • Consulting
www.cr-eatingbalance.com

Library of Congress
ISBN-13: 978-0-9790820-0-9
ISBN-10: 0-9790820-0-5

Printed in the United States of America

To Dane, Simone and Blake

Disclaimer

The information, scientific studies, specific solutions and opinions discussed, while carefully researched, are offered for educational purposes only. They are not intended as a diagnoses or treatment for any specific ailment, or a replacement for the expertise of your qualified healthcare provider.

Diet can have a profound impact on how people experience disease and is a powerful tool for disease prevention. Although many foods have reported medical benefits, if you have any type of health problem or physical symptoms, do not self diagnose or self treat—even with a food or herb.

The information in this publication is based on the most current nutritional data available at the time of publication. Product formulations and Ingredients may change. And actual nutrition values may differ slightly due to product preparation.

Food/Product sources include the USDA National Nutrient Database for Standard Reference, Release 19, product NUTRITION FACTS labels and INGREDIENTS lists. Data extracted from the USDA National Nutrient Database for Standard Reference, Release 19 has been rounded to the nearest whole number.

Generic and brand name product information is available throughout this guide. At this time, the USDA does not provide "INGREDIENT" lists for foods/products referenced in the USDA National Nutrient Database for Standard Reference, Release 19; and therefore, Ingredient information is not available for generic products. Brand name foods/products have been fully researched and documented. "na" has been used in the listings to indicate when nutrition information was "not available" for a specific item.

For the most current information about food products, check the NUTRITION FACTS label and INGREDIENTS list prior to purchase.

The author and/or publisher do not represent or receive compensation of any kind from food products/manufacturers listed in this book. The author and/or publisher are not responsible for typographical errors. If you believe an error has been made or would like to see one or more products or brands highlighted in this guide, please contact us via our website at:

www.cr-eatingbalance.com

eating smart \ēt'ing • smärt\ *vb* **1**: a paradigm shift from the way you value food **2**: moving from quantity to quality **3**: balancing healthy food and your favorite food becomes a way of life.

"Adopting healthy behaviors such as eating nutritious foods, being physically active, and avoiding tobacco use can prevent or control the devastating effects of heart disease, cancer and diabetes."

— **Center for Disease Control and Prevention**

Contents

Introduction — *9*

How to Use This Guide — *10*
Daily Servings Simplified *10*
Two Types of Food *12*
Percent Daily Values *13*
Ingredients Decoded *17*
    Artificial Sweeteners *18*
    High Fructose Corn Syrup *19*
    Hydrogenated Fat *19*
    Partially Hydrogenated Oils (Trans Fat) *19*
    Whole and Enriched Grains *20*
What are Organics? *22*

The Fruit Group — *24*
    Fruit and Fruit Juices *26*

The Vegetables Group — *34*
    Vegetables and Vegetable Juices *36*

The Grain Group — *50*
Breads and Cereals *52*
    Breads and Crackers *54*
    Cereals *60*
    Pancakes, Pastries and Waffles *66*
Grains, Pasta and Rice *70*
    Grains *72*
    Pasta *72*
    Rice *80*

The Meat and Bean Group — *82*
Dry Beans, Peas and Tofu *84*
Nuts, Nut Butters and Seeds *92*
Beef, Pork and Lamb *100*
    Beef *102*
    Lamb and Goat *106*
    Pork *106*
Lunch Meats, Sausage and Franks *114*
    Lunch Meats *116*
    Sausage and Franks *118*

Contents *continued*

Poultry—Chicken, Duck, Goose and Turkey ... *122*
    Chicken *124*
    Duck and Goose *128*
    Turkey *128*
Fish and Shellfish *132*
    Fish *134*
    Shellfish *144*
Eggs *148*

The Milk Group — *152*
    Milk *154*
    Yogurt *156*
    Cheese *160*

Oils — *168*
    Oils *170*

Discretionary or Optional Choices — *174*
Dairy and Non-Dairy *176*
    Dairy *178*
    Non Dairy *180*
Buttermilk, Lard, Margarine and Shortening ... *184*
Condiments, Salad Dressing and Mayonnaise ... *190*
    Condiments *192*
    Salad Dressings *198*
    Mayonnaise *204*
Herbs, Spices, Salt and Seasonings *206*
Sauces, Gravies and Marinades *214*
    Sauces *216*
    Gravy and Marinades *218*
Jelly, Jams, Sweeteners and Syrup *222*
    Jelly and Jams *224*
    Sugar and Sweeteners *226*
    Syrup *228*
Soups *232*

Codes and Abbreviations — *242*
References — *244*
About the Author — *247*

Introduction

Food is a powerful tool for disease prevention, yet millions of Americans don't understand nutrition. Is it the conflicting information, complicated servings sizes or the infamous "Ingredients list" filled with scientific terms only a chemist can decipher?

Eating healthy doesn't mean you have to deprive yourself of your favorite foods—if you eat smart.

Are the Blueberries in Your Waffles Really Blueberries?™ was created to guide you through the complex world of nutrition and help you focus on what's really important; and it's easier than you think. The three basics are—what to eat, how much and how to locate the best products available.

Are the Blueberries in Your Waffles Really Blueberries?™ is the only guide to highlight products high in fat, saturated fat, sodium and fiber, which are the foundation for a healthy life. In addition, it goes one step further by covering Ingredients, the key to understanding the true quality of food; making this an indispensable comparison guide and resource for eating healthy.

Substantially increase your knowledge about food and nutrition. When you finally understand where you need to focus, you're less likely to be swayed by the latest study or compelling marketing. You can make better choices at the grocery store or when dining-out. Eating healthy becomes a way of life.

How to Use This Guide

Daily Servings Simplified

There are five main food groups defined by the United States Department of Agriculture (USDA):

Fruits
Vegetables
Grains
Meat and Beans
Milk

The USDA recommends eating "servings" from each of the five food groups daily. A "serving" can mean many things to different people. Is a serving one ounce, one cup or a plate full?

For example: The USDA suggests eating 6 to 11 "servings" of Grains per day and 2 to 3 "servings" from the Meat and Bean Group, which leaves a lot of room for interpretation.

The USDA has developed a website which helps eliminates these potential misinterpretations. Instead of saying "6 to 11" servings of Grains per day, it now says eat one "six ounce serving." The serving for the Meat and Beans Group is 5.5 ounces.

The USDA converted all Daily Servings to this simple format. Page 11 has an example of servings sizes simplified for each of the food groups, based on a 2,000 calorie diet.

Nutrition facts on food labels are **always** based on a 2,000 calorie diet. Therefore, a 2,000 calorie diet is the baseline for information used throughout this guide. This established amount is based on the "average person" who needs 2,000 calories each day to stay healthy.

Your caloric needs may be higher or lower. For your personalized "serving" results go to **www.mypyramid.gov** or **www.cr-eatingbalance.com**.

Example:

Fruits	2 cups
Vegetables	2.5 cups
Grains	6 ounces
Meat and Beans	5.5 ounces
Milk	3 cups

Many different types of food can fall into one of the five main food groups. For example, the Grain Group includes breads, cereals, crackers, rice and pasta, etc., while the Meat and Beans Group includes meat, poultry, fish, dry beans and peas, nuts and seeds.

Notice the serving recommendation listed above for the Grain Group is six ounces. A three ounce serving is equal to the size of a deck of cards. Two decks of cards lying side by side or stacked are comparable to a six ounce serving. Six ounces is the total amount of Grains (breads, cereals, crackers, rice and pasta, etc.) to be consumed in one day.

Visualizing a **deck of cards** when you eat foods from the Grain Group or Meat and Beans Group is helpful at home and when dining-out. For the other food groups, imagine the size of a **baseball** which is equivalent to one cup. This will help to better manage the amount of food you eat in one sitting.

Vegetarians may exclude some or all animal derived foods from their eating plan (which could include meat, eggs, and/or dairy products). Substitutes for these foods or food groups are available and a nutritionally balanced diet can be achieved. The following nutrients need particular attention: protein, iron, vitamin B-12, vitamin D and calcium.

Two Types of Food

Basically, there are two types of foods—**plant** and **animal** foods. When you grasp this simple concept, making good food choices becomes easier.

Plant foods are fruits, vegetables, grains, dry beans and peas, nuts and seeds. Essentially, any type of food that comes from a plant. When you think about "plant" foods think **carbohydrates**.

Most carbohydrates come from plant-based foods. Carbohydrates include: sugar, fiber and starch. Dairy products (milk, cheese etc.) are the only animal foods containing a significant amount of carbohydrates, due to the natural sugar or "lactose" found in milk.

Plant foods **do not contain cholesterol** and **only plant foods contain fiber,** a vital nutrient for good health. A high-fiber diet can help lower your risk of heart disease, cancer and diabetes.

Take a moment to look at "The Fruit Group" beginning on page 26. Notice the nutrients columns at the top of the page. Locate the Cholesterol column and quickly glance down the list of fruit and fruit juices. The entire column shows "0" for cholesterol. Fruit (a plant food) does not contain cholesterol. And as you will see, all fruits, except avocados, contain no fat or saturated fat.

On the other hand, the Carbohydrate, Fiber, and Sugar columns are filled with information.

All **animal** derived products such as meat, fish, poultry, dairy, eggs etc. **contain fat, saturated fat and cholesterol.** The amount varies depending on the product.

Turn to "The Beef, Pork and Lamb" chapter on page 100. Note the Total Fat, Saturated Fat and Cholesterol columns are filled with information, while most of the Carbohydrate, Fiber and Sugar columns list "0". If you look further down the list, you'll notice products containing carbohydrates. In most cases, this is due to sugar or flour (a plant-based food) being added to a product.

Labeling fresh meat, poultry and fish is optional. So odds are you won't find details about fat, saturated fat and cholesterol content for most of these foods at your local grocery store.

Get the facts, for fresh meat, poultry and fish, in this guide prior to shopping. You may be surprised just how much fat you can eliminate by choosing a different cut or grade of meat. This is what eating smart is all about.

Let's recap: 1) Plant foods contain carbohydrates. They have zero cholesterol and only plant foods contain fiber. 2) Animal foods contain fat, saturated fat and cholesterol; most do not contain carbohydrates (sugar, fiber and starch). Keep this in mind as we continue to move forward.

Percent Daily Values

The basic guidelines for eating healthy are 1) eat foods low in fat, especially saturated fat, trans fat and cholesterol; 2) avoid high levels of sodium; and 3) get plenty of fiber.

One easy way to balance these nutrients is to reference Percent (%) Daily Values. Percent (%) Daily Values are the percentage of nutrients (fat, saturated fat, trans fat, cholesterol, sodium, fiber, etc.) in a serving of food.

Percent (%) Daily Values are found on a NUTRITION FACTS label. NUTRITION FACTS labels can be found on most packaged food and are also available online or upon request at most deli's, restaurants and fast food establishments.

You can use Percent (%) Daily Values as a quick reference for managing daily intake of nutrients essential for healthy eating. This is an excellent tool for comparing foods to see which ones are lowest in fat or high in fiber.

Nutrition Facts

Serving Size 1 Cup (228g)
Servings Per Container 2

Amount Per Serving

Calories 250   Calories from Fat 110

% Daily Value*

Total Fat 12g	18%
Saturated Fat 3g	15%
Trans Fat 3g	
Cholesterol 30mg	10%
Sodium 470mg	20%
Total Carbohydrate 31g	10%
Dietary Fiber 0g	0%
Sugars 5g	
Protein 5g	
Vitamin A	4%
Vitamin C	2%
Calcium	20%
Iron	4%

* Percent Daily Values are based on a 2,000 calorie diet. Your Daily Values may be higher or lower depending on your calorie needs.

	Calories:	2,000	2,500
Total Fat	Less than	65g	80g
Sat Fat	Less than	20g	25g
Cholesterol	Less than	300mg	300mg
Sodium	Less than	2,400mg	2,400mg
Total Carbohydrate		300g	375g
Dietary Fiber		25g	30g

☐ **% Daily Value :** 5% or less is Low
　　　　　　　　　　20% or more is High

☐ **Limit these Nutrients**

☐ **Get Enough of these Nutrients**

☐ **Footnote**

Example is colored for demonstration purposes only.

1. A % Daily Value column found on the far right side of the NUTRITON FACTS label.
2. The Center for Food Safety and Applied Nutrition (CFSAN) suggests **5% or less of a nutrient is low and 20% or more is high.**
3. **Limit** nutrients such as fat, saturated fat, Trans Fats, cholesterol and sodium. While some of these nutrients are necessary (in small amounts), over consumption is a root cause of disease.
4. Be sure to **Get Enough** fiber, vitamins and minerals. Remember only plant foods contain fiber.

   Look at the NUTRITION FACTS example provided. Notice the % Daily Value column on the right hand side. Sodium's % Daily Value is 20%, meaning this product is high in a nutrient that needs to be limited. The serving size in the NUTRITION FACTS example is 1 cup. If you eat two cups, then you'll need to double the amount of sodium (and all other nutrients). You've now consumed 40%. If you eat five one cup servings, you've just consumed 100% of a days worth of sodium (20 x 5 servings = 100).

5. A **Footnote** may be provided at the bottom of the NUTRITION FACTS label outlining the recommended % Daily Value for total fat, saturated fat, cholesterol, sodium, carbohydrates and fiber.

   Note: The FDA has not established a % Daily Value for Trans Fats, sugar or protein.

   Footnote verbiage such as "Less than" indicates limiting nutrients such as fat, saturated fat, cholesterol and sodium. Take time to look at each of the recommendations located in the Footnote: Eat "Less than" 65 grams (g) of Total Fat per day, "Less than" 20 grams (g) of Saturated fat, and so on. This is your guideline for healthy eating.

As a reminder to **limit** nutrients such as fat, saturated fat, Trans Fats, cholesterol and sodium each of their nutrient columns throughout this guide will be **highlighted in grey.**

The Fiber column will be **highlighted in green,** a cue to **"Get Enough"** of this nutrient.

The symbol ↑ will be used when foods/products are **high** in nutrients **(20% or more)** such as fat, saturated fat, cholesterol, sodium and fiber.

If the symbol ↑ falls into the Fiber column, this is a good sign. Choose products high in fiber more often.

If the symbol ↑ appears in the Fat, Saturated Fat, Cholesterol or Sodium column of any given product, look for another similar product lower in the applicable nutrient, reduce your serving size or simply watch your intake for the rest of the day. These are nutrients we need to limit; balance is key.

A % Daily Value has not been set for Trans Fat. You will not see the symbol ↑ in the Trans Fat column to call out foods/products high in this nutrient; however, the column is highlighted in grey as a reminder to limit Trans Fat. Zero Trans Fat is best.

Example:

Item	Serving	Cal	Total Fat (g)	Sat Fat (g)	Trans Fat (g)
Avocado					
California, all varieties	½ fruit	114	10	1	0
Florida, all varieties	½ fruit	182	↑15	3	0

Ingredients Decoded

Reviewing a product's INGREDIENTS list will help you determine the overall quality and potential health benefit of any given product.

Are the blueberries in your waffles really blueberries, or are they artificial blueberry flavored bits?

Does your "heart healthy" margarine contain heart damaging Trans Fats? The answers to these questions can only be found in the INGREDIENTS list.

Ingredient lists are required on labels of foods with more than one Ingredient. Ingredients are listed in descending order of weight.

Example:

> **INGREDIENTS:** WHOLE WHEAT FLOUR, HIGH FRUCTOSE CORN SYRUP, PARTIALLY HYDROGENATED SOYBEAN AND/OR COTTONSEED OIL, MILK PROTEIN CONCENTRATE, SALT, YELLOW 5, YELLOW 6.

Whole wheat flour is the first Ingredient on the INGREDIENTS list; therefore, this product's main or primary Ingredient is whole wheat flour. Yellow 6 (an artificial color) is the last Ingredient meaning less was used.

Chol (mg)	Sod (mg)	Carb (mg)	Fiber (g)	Sugar (g)	Prot (g)
0	5	6	↑5	0	1
0	3	12	↑9	4	3

The INGREDIENTS list can be intimidating filled with scientific chemical terms that many of us choose to ignore, either consciously or unconsciously. We're often drawn to our favorite brand or focus on the fat or carbohydrate content and not so much what's in the product.

If a product's INGREDIENTS list is filled with more chemical Ingredients than recognizable Ingredients that are actually food, you may want to keep looking. There are many similar products out there—many choices, healthier choices.

To save you time and to help you compare the quality of a product, this guide highlights the six top Ingredients found in hundreds of foods/products many people look for or avoid, either for personal or health related reasons.

1. Artificial Sweeteners
2. High Fructose Corn Syrup
3. Hydrogenated Fat
4. Partially Hydrogenated Oils (Trans Fat)
5. Whole Grains
6. Enriched Grains

Artificial Sweeteners

Artificial Sweeteners can be useful when used appropriately for people with diabetes who need to control their sugar intake. Artificial Sweeteners are low in calories and do not affect blood sugar levels.

Natural alternatives for Artificial Sweeteners include stevia and agave nectar. Both have a low Glycemic rating and are considered safe for diabetics. A Glycemic rating or the Glycemic Index (GI) is a ranking system for carbohydrates and the effect on our blood sugar (glucose) level. Please check with your health care provider before making changes to your diet.

Keep your eyes on total calories consumed. Artificial Sweeteners are not a free ticket to eat more.

High Fructose Corn Syrup

High Fructose Corn Syrup (HFCS) is a sweetener and preservative used to extend the shelf life of many processed foods. HFCS is made from corn and is sweeter and less expensive than table sugar. The "added" sweetness in HFCS may actually stimulate the appetite.

High Fructose Corn Syrup is found in almost all sugar-based soft drinks. It is also found in fruit juice, canned fruit, flavored milk, breads and baked products, condiments and many other processed foods often high in calories and low in nutrition. It is best to limit these types of foods.

Hydrogenated Fat

Hydrogenation is the chemical process used to turn liquid vegetable oil into a solid fat i.e. shortening or stick margarine. Hydrogenated Fats are high in saturated fat (your artery clogging fats) and should be limited.

Partially Hydrogenated Oils

Partially Hydrogenated Oils contain Trans Fats. Trans Fats not only raise your total cholesterol, they deplete good cholesterol, which protects us against heart disease.

Trans Fats are found in every food that has "partially hydrogenated" followed by a vegetable oil, such as soybean, cottonseed oil etc.

on the INGREDIENTS list. Small amounts of Trans Fats are also found in animal products such as full fat dairy and beef.

"Zero Trans Fat per serving."

The Food and Drug Administration (FDA) allows foods containing less than 0.5 grams of Trans Fat per serving, to be listed on the package's NUTRITION FACTS label as "0g." When a label shows 0 grams of Trans Fat and lists "partially hydrogenated" oil, the product may contain up to 0.49 grams of Trans Fat per serving. This can quickly add up.

The words "per serving" are an indicator the product contains Trans Fat.

Although a Daily Value has not been set for Trans Fat, the suggested intake is less than 1% of your total daily calories. If you consume 2,000 calories a day, that works out to two grams (one fat gram equals nine calories) of Trans Fat or less.

Always read the INGREDIENTS list. Avoid products containing Partially Hydrogenated Oil, regardless of where it is listed on the INGREDIENTS list. Zero Trans Fat is best.

Whole and Enriched Grains

Grains are the seeds of plants. Whole grains include the entire seed, the germ, bran and endosperm. The bran and germ of the seed contain high amounts of fiber and essential nutrients.

Refined grains have been milled, a process that removes the bran, germ, fiber and nutrients. White flour and wheat flour are examples of refined grains. Refined grains are considered to be poor in nutrition.

Enriched grains are refined grains "enriched" with vitamins lost in the milling process; however, fiber and various other B vitamins are not added back.

Most grains are refined grains and therefore are not highlighted in this guide unless they are "mixed" with Whole or Enriched Grains.

Eat foods/products containing Whole Grains more often.

EAT SMART:

Products containing **Artificial Sweeteners** are identified with an [A] under the Sugar column throughout this guide.

Products with **High Fructose Corn Syrup** are identified with an [HF] under the Sugar column throughout this guide.

Hydrogenated Fats are identified with an [H] under the Trans Fat column throughout this guide.

Partially Hydrogenated Oils are identified with a [P] under the Trans Fat column throughout this guide.

Whole Grains are identified with a [W] under the Fiber column throughout this guide.

Enriched Grains, which are also refined grains, are identified with an [E] in the Fiber column throughout this guide.

Products that contain a **mix of Whole Grains and Enriched Grains** are identified with a [W] and [E] throughout this guide.

Products containing a **mix of Whole Grains and refined grains** are identified with a [W] and [R] throughout this guide.

What are Organics?

Organic products continue to grow in popularity. When asked, consumers are choosing Organic over conventional products primarily to reduce pesticide consumption. Organic products offer much more than a reduction in pesticides. There are six key components defining Organics and three levels of Organic products available. **For a free quick reference Organic Wallet Guide go to:**

www.cr-eatingbalance.com

---

or·gan·ic (ôr-găn' ĭk)
Organic meat, poultry, eggs, and dairy products come from animals that are given no antibiotics or growth hormones. Organic food is produced without using most conventional pesticides, fertilizers made with synthetic ingredients or sewage sludge, bioengineering, or ionizing radiation.

— **USDA National Organic Program**

A high fiber diet can help lower your risk of heart disease, cancer and diabetes.

Only plant foods contain fiber.

The Fruit Group

Fruit and Fruit Juices

USDA Recommendations:

Eat a variety of fruit.

Choose fresh, frozen, canned or dried fruit.

Go easy on fruit juices.

KEEP IT SIMPLE

Eat 2 cups per day.
USDA recommended Daily Serving is based on a 2,000 calorie diet.

Fruit and all plant foods (carbohydrates) **contain fiber.** A high-fiber diet can help lower your risk of heart disease, cancer and diabetes.

Fruit does not contain cholesterol and is naturally **low in fat and saturated fat.** An exception is the avocado which is high in "healthy fat." Compare California and Florida avocados in this chapter. Notice California varieties are lower in fat than Florida avocados; however, Florida varieties are ↑ in fiber. Both are excellent choices due to the "healthy fat." Smaller servings are recommended since fat is a nutrient that needs to be limited.

Fruit naturally contains sugar and is **low in sodium.**

Canned or processed fruit or fruit juices may contain added sweeteners such as sugar, corn syrup, High Fructose Corn Syrup or Artificial Sweeteners.

Many fruit juices and other fruit beverages are high in sugar. Go easy on these beverages especially those with added sweeteners.

Canned products labeled "in heavy syrup" usually contain High Fructose Corn Syrup or corn syrup.

EAT SMART. To reduce added sweeteners in fruit, look for canned fruit packed in "natural" juices, or eat fresh or frozen fruit. Some "fruit juices" are more like fruit flavored beverages. They contain little to no real fruit. Look for fruit juices labeled as "100% fruit juice."

Item	Serving	Cal	Total Fat (g)	Sat Fat (g)	Trans Fat (g)
FRUIT and FRUIT JUICES					
Apple					
Fresh, with skin	1 med	72	0	0	0
Fresh, without skin	1 med	61	0	0	0
Juice, unsweetened	1 cup	117	0	0	0
Applesauce					
Sweetened, Motts®	1 cup	100	0	0	0
Unsweetened, Motts®, Natural	1 cup	50	0	0	0
Apricot					
Fresh	1 fruit	17	0	0	0
Dried	½ cup	8	0	0	0
Juice, R.W. Knudsen®, nectar	1 cup	130	0	0	0
Avocado					
California, all varieties	½ fruit	114	10	1	0
Florida, all varieties	½ fruit	182	↑15	3	0
Banana					
Fresh – 7"	1 med	105	0	0	0
Blueberries					
Fresh	½ cup	42	0	0	0
Frozen, Cascadian Farms®, Organic	½ cup	35	0	0	0
Canned, Oregon®, in lite syrup	½ cup	110	0	0	0
Juice, R.W. Knudsen®, Just Blueberry	1 cup	100	0	0	0
Cantaloupe					
Fresh, diced	1 cup	53	0	0	0
Cranberries					
Fresh, whole berries	½ cup	22	0	0	0
Dried, Ocean Spray®, Craisens	⅓ cup	130	0	0	0
Juice, Ocean Spray®	8 oz	130	0	0	0
Juice, sweetened	1 cup	137	0	0	0
Juice, unsweetened	1 cup	116	0	0	0
Cherries					
Fresh, Sweet, no pits	½ cup	46	0	0	0

Chol (mg)	Sod (mg)	Carb (g)	Fiber (g)	Sugar (g)	Prot (g)
0	0	19	3	14	0
0	0	16	2	13	0
0	7	30	0	27	0
0	0	24	1	22 HF	0
0	0	12	1	11	0
0	0	4	1	3	0
0	0	2	0	2	0
0	30	30	0	26	1
0	5	6	↑5	0	1
0	3	12	↑9	4	3
0	1	27	3	14	1
0	1	11	2	7	0
0	0	9	2	6	0
0	5	26	2	18	0
0	10	24	0	18	0
0	25	13	1	12	1
0	2	6	2	2	0
0	0	33	2	27	0
0	35	33	0	33 HF	0
0	5	34	0	30	0
0	5	31	0	31	1
0	0	12	2	9	1

Fruit and Fruit Juices | 27

Item	Serving	Cal	Total Fat (g)	Sat Fat (g)	Trans Fat (g)
Cherries *continued*					
Frozen, Cascadian Farms®, Sweet Cherries, Organic	1 cup	90	0	0	0
Canned, Sweet, in heavy syrup, no pits	½ cup	75	0	0	0
Jar, Mezzetta®, Maraschino	1 cherry	10	0	0	0
Juice, R.W. Knudsen®, Just Tart	1 cup	130	0	0	0
Fig					
Fresh – 2¼"	1 med	37	0	0	0
Dried	1 fruit	21	0	0	0
Fruit Drinks					
SunnyD®, Original Citrus drink	8 oz	120	0	0	0
SunnyD®, Fruit Punch	8 oz	120	0	0	0
Grapes					
Fresh, red or green	9 grapes	34	0	0	0
Juice, Old Orchard®, frozen concentrate	8 oz	160	0	0	0
Goji					
Dried, berries, Himalania®, Organic	1 oz	150	0	0	0
Juice, Pure Fruit Technologies™, Goji-Zen	1 oz	15	0	0	0
Honeydew					
Fresh, diced	1 cup	61	0	0	0
Kiwifruit					
Fresh	1 med	46	0	0	0
Lemon					
Fresh, with peel	1 fruit	22	0	0	0
Fresh, without peel	1 fruit	24	0	0	0
Juice, Lemon	1 tbsp	3	0	0	0
Peel, Lemon (zest)	1 tbsp	3	0	0	0
Lemonade, Capri Sun®	1 pouch	100	0	0	0
Lemonade, Minute Maid®	8 oz	100	0	0	0

Chol (mg)	Sod (mg)	Carb (g)	Fiber (g)	Sugar (g)	Prot (g)
0	0	22	3	18	1
0	2	19	2	17	1
0	0	2	0	2 HF	1
0	30	32	0	24	1
0	0	10	1	8	0
0	1	5	1	4	0
0	190	29	0	27 HF	0
0	160	29	0	28 HF	0
0	1	9	0	8	0
0	20	42	0	40	0
0	190	32	1	30	5
0	0	4	0	3	0
0	31	15	1	14	1
0	2	11	2	7	1
0	3	12	↑5	na	1
0	2	8	2	2	1
0	0	1	0	0	0
0	0	1	1	0	0
0	15	27	0	27 HF	0
0	35	28	0	27 HF	0

Fruit and Fruit Juices

Item	Serving	Cal	Total Fat (g)	Sat Fat (g)	Trans Fat (g)
Mango					
Fresh, sliced	½ cup	107	0	0	0
Noni					
Juice, Pure Fruit Technologies™, Hawaiian Noni	2 tbsp	15	0	0	0
Orange					
Fresh – 2⅝"	1 med	62	0	0	0
Juice, frozen concentrate	1 cup	112	0	0	0
Pomegranate					
Fresh	1 fruit	105	0	0	0
Juice, R.W. Knudsen®, unsweetened	1 cup	150	0	0	0
Papaya					
Fresh, cubes	½ cup	27	0	0	0
Peach					
Fresh – 2⅔"	1 med	58	0	0	0
Canned, halves, in heavy syrup	1 half	56	0	0	0
Canned, halves, in lite syrup	1 half	53	0	0	0
Canned, sliced, Del Monte®, Carb Clever™	½ cup	39	0	0	0
Pear					
Fresh	1 med	103	0	0	0
Canned, chunks, Del Monte®, Carb Clever™	½ cup	40	0	0	0
Canned, halves, in heavy syrup	1 half	56	0	0	0
Canned, halves, in lite syrup	1 half	43	0	0	0
Pineapple					
Fresh, all varieties, sliced	½ cup	37	0	0	0
Canned, in heavy syrup, chunks	½ cup	99	0	0	0
Canned, in lite syrup, chunks	½ cup	66	0	0	0
Juice, unsweetened	1 cup	132	0	0	0
Juice, R.W. Knudsen®, Organic	1 cup	120	0	0	0

Chol (mg)	Sod (mg)	Carb (g)	Fiber (g)	Sugar (g)	Prot (g)
0	3	28	2	24	1
0	0	4	0	3	0
0	0	15	3	12	1
0	2	27	1	21	2
0	5	26	1	26	1
0	20	38	0	36	0
0	4	7	1	4	0
0	0	14	2	13	1
0	4	14	2	13	0
0	5	14	1	13	0
0	10	7	1	6 [A]	1
0	2	28	↑6	17	1
0	10	10	1	9 [A]	0
0	4	15	1	12	0
0	4	12	1	9	0
0	1	1	1	7	0
0	3	26	1	22	0
0	3	17	1	16	0
0	5	32	0	25	1
0	15	28	0	28	0

Fruit and Fruit Juices

Item	Serving	Cal	Total Fat (g)	Sat Fat (g)	Trans Fat (g)
Plum					
Fresh	1 fruit	30	0	0	0
Raspberries					
Fresh	10	10	0	0	0
Raisins					
Dried, seedless	Sm. box	129	0	0	0
Dried, Sun-Made®, Organic, seedless	1.5 oz box	130	0	0	0
Strawberries					
Fresh, whole	½ cup	23	0	0	0
Tangerine (mandarin oranges)					
Raw – 2½"	1 med	47	0	0	0
Canned in lite syrup	½ cup	77	0	0	0
Watermelon					
Fresh, diced	1 cup	46	0	0	0
Fruit Cocktail					
Canned, Del Monte® Carb Clever™	½ cup	40	0	0	0
Canned, in heavy syrup, drained	½ cup	75	0	0	0
Canned, in lite syrup	½ cup	69	0	0	0

Chol (mg)	Sod (mg)	Carb (g)	Fiber (g)	Sugar (g)	Prot (g)
0	0	8	1	7	0
0	0	2	1	1	0
0	10	34	2	25	1
0	10	33	2	30	1
0	1	5	2	4	0
0	2	12	2	9	1
0	15	20	1	20	1
0	2	11	1	9	1
0	10	11	0	10 [A]	9
0	13	20	2	19	1
0	7	18	1	17	0

The Vegetable Group

Vegetables and Vegetable Juices

USDA Recommendations:

Eat more dark green vegetables.

Eat more orange vegetables.

KEEP IT SIMPLE

Eat 2.5 cups per day.
USDA recommended Daily Serving is based on a 2,000 calorie diet.

Vegetables and all plant foods (carbohydrates) **contain fiber.** A high-fiber diet can help lower your risk of heart disease, cancer and diabetes.

Vegetables **do not contain cholesterol** and are naturally **low in fat, saturated fat, sodium** and sugar.

Canned or processed vegetables may be ↑ in **sodium.** Go to the "Peppers" in this chapter. Notice, raw jalapenos have "0" sodium. The other three canned jalapeno's sodium content varies quite a bit. One is ↑ in sodium, while a different brand has 30mg. Selecting the product with only 30mg is a smart choice— a potential savings of 550mg of sodium. Take time to compare the sodium content in all canned vegetables.

Boxed or frozen vegetables with cheese or cream based sauces, and many boxed or frozen potatoes, contain **Trans Fats.** Look at the products coded with a [P] in this chapter. These products contain Trans Fats (partially hydrogenated oils) and should be avoided.

EAT SMART. To reduce sodium look for low sodium or "no salt added" canned products or eat fresh or frozen vegetables. Lessen fat by purchasing plain products and add your own low fat toppings, including low fat cheese and sauces, use fresh herbs or Trans Fat free spreads.

VEGETABLES and VEGETABLE JUICES

Item	Serving	Cal	Total Fat (g)	Sat Fat (g)	Trans Fat (g)
Artichokes					
Raw, whole	1 med	6	0	0	0
Frozen, cooked, no salt	1 cup	76	0	0	0
Marinated, hearts, Maria®	2 pieces	25	0	0	0
Asparagus					
Raw	4 spears	16	0	0	0
Frozen	4 spears	14	0	0	0
Canned	4 spears	12	0	0	0
Bamboo Shoots					
Raw	1 cup	41	0	0	0
Canned	1 cup	25	1	0	0
Beans, Green					
Raw	½ cup	17	0	0	0
Frozen	½ cup	20	0	0	0
Canned, with salt	½ cup	18	0	0	0
Canned, no salt	½ cup	18	0	0	0
Broccoli					
Raw, chopped	½ cup	15	0	0	0
Frozen	½ cup	20	0	0	0
Brussels Sprouts					
Raw	½ cup	19	0	0	0
Cabbage					
Chinese, raw, shredded	1 cup	9	0	0	0
Common, raw, shredded	½ cup	8	0	0	0
Red, raw, shredded	½ cup	11	0	0	0
Savoy, raw shredded	½ cup	9	0	0	0
Cardoon					
Raw	½ cup	15	0	0	0
Carrot					
Raw, chopped	½ cup	26	0	0	0
Frozen, chopped	½ cup	23	0	0	0
Canned, sliced	½ cup	18	0	0	0

Chol (mg)	Sod (mg)	Carb (g)	Fiber (g)	Sugar (g)	Prot (g)
0	120	13	↑7	0	4
0	89	15	↑8	1	5
0	105	3	1	0	1
0	0	3	1	1	1
0	5	2	1	0	2
0	52	2	1	1	2
0	6	8	3	5	4
0	9	4	2	2	2
0	4	4	2	1	1
0	2	5	2	0	1
0	311	4	2	0	1
0	17	4	2	0	1
0	15	3	1	1	1
0	19	4	2	1	2
0	11	4	2	1	1
0	46	2	1	1	1
0	6	2	1	0	0
0	9	3	1	1	1
0	10	2	1	1	1
0	151	4	1	0	1
0	44	6	2	3	0
0	44	5	2	3	1
0	177	4	1	2	0

Vegetables and Vegetable Juices

Item	Serving	Cal	Total Fat (g)	Sat Fat (g)	Trans Fat (g)
Carrot continued					
Juice, canned	½ cup	94	0	0	0
Cauliflower					
Raw	½ cup	12	0	0	0
Celery					
Raw, med stalk 7½" – 8"	1 stalk	6	0	0	0
Celeriac					
Raw	½ cup	33	0	0	0
Chard					
Raw	½ cup	3	0	0	0
Collards					
Raw	½ cup	5	0	0	0
Corn					
Raw, yellow sweet, 6¾" – 7½"	1 med ear	77	1	0	0
Frozen, yellow sweet, kernels	½ cup	72	0	0	0
Cucumber					
Raw, with peel	½ cup	8	0	0	0
Raw, no peel	½ cup	7	0	0	0
Dandelion Greens					
Raw	½ cup	12	0	0	0
Edamame (soybean pods)					
Frozen, Cascadian Farms®, Organic	⅔ cup	120	5	0	0
Eggplant					
Raw, with peel	¼ plant	33	0	0	0
Raw, no peel	¼ plant	27	0	0	0
Endive					
Raw, chopped	½ cup	4	0	0	0
Fennel					
Raw	1 bulb	73	0	0	0
Garlic					
Raw	1 clove	4	0	0	0

Vegetables and Vegetable Juices

Chol (mg)	Sod (mg)	Carb (g)	Fiber (g)	Sugar (g)	Prot (g)
0	68	22	2	9	2
0	15	3	1	1	1
0	32	1	1	1	0
0	78	7	1	1	1
0	38	1	0	0	0
0	4	1	1	0	0
0	14	17	2	3	3
0	2	17	2	3	2
0	1	2	0	1	0
0	1	1	0	1	0
0	21	3	1	1	1
0	10	9	3	2	10
0	3	8	↑5	3	1
0	2	7	4	3	1
0	6	0	0	0	0
0	122	17	↑7	0	3
0	1	1	0	0	0

Vegetables and Vegetable Juices

Item	Serving	Cal	Total Fat (g)	Sat Fat (g)	Trans Fat (g)
Jicama (yam bean)					
Raw, sliced	½ cup	25	0	0	0
Kale					
Raw	½ cup	17	0	0	0
Kohlrabi					
Raw	½ cup	18	0	0	0
Leek					
Raw, lower leaf	1 leek	54	0	0	0
Lettuce					
Boston/Bibb	1 cup	7	0	0	0
Greenleaf	1 cup	5	0	0	0
Iceberg	1 cup	10	0	0	0
Romaine	1 cup	8	0	0	0
Mixed Vegetables					
Frozen, Green Giant®	⅔ cup	50	0	0	0
Canned	½ cup	40	0	0	0
Mushrooms					
Canned	¼ cup	10	0	0	0
Green Giant®, jar	½ cup	25	0	0	0
Portabella, raw	¼ cup	6	0	0	0
Shiitake, dried	4	44	0	0	0
White, raw	¼ cup	4	0	0	0
Mustard Greens					
Raw	½ cup	7	0	0	0
Okra					
Raw	½ cup	16	0	0	0
Onions					
Dehydrated	1 tbsp	17	0	0	0
Onions, raw	½ cup	32	0	0	0
Sweet, raw	½ onion	53	0	0	0
Pea Pods (snow peas)					
Raw, whole	½ cup	13	0	0	0
Peas					
Raw	½ cup	59	0	0	0
Frozen	½ cup	55	0	0	0
Canned	½ cup	59	0	0	0

Chol (mg)	Sod (mg)	Carb (g)	Fiber (g)	Sugar (g)	Prot (g)
0	3	6	3	1	0
0	14	3	1	0	1
0	14	4	2	2	1
0	18	13	2	3	1
0	3	1	1	1	1
0	10	1	0	0	0
0	7	2	1	1	0
0	4	2	1	1	0
0	20	11	2	3	2
0	121	8	2	2	2
0	166	2	1	1	1
0	440	4	1	1	2
0	1	1	0	0	1
0	2	11	2	0	1
0	1	1	0	0	1
0	7	1	1	0	1
0	4	4	2	0	1
0	1	4	0	2	0
0	3	7	1	3	1
0	13	13	2	8	1
0	1	2	1	1	1
0	4	10	4	4	4
0	81	10	3	4	4
0	214	11	4	4	4

Vegetables and Vegetable Juices

Item	Serving	Cal	Total Fat (g)	Sat Fat (g)	Trans Fat (g)
Peppers					
Chili, green, Macayo® diced, canned	2 tbsp	5	0	0	0
Green, sweet, raw, 2¾" – 2½"	1 med	24	0	0	0
Jalapeno, raw	1	4	0	0	0
Jalapeno, canned	1	6	0	0	0
Jalapeno, La Costena®, sliced, canned	3 tbsp	5	0	0	0
Jalapeno, Macayo's®, diced, canned	2 tbsp	10	0	0	0
Red, sweet, raw, 2¾" – 2½"	1 med	31	0	0	0
Yellow, sweet, raw	1	50	0	0	0
Potatoes					
Au Gratin, Betty Crocker®, dry mix, prepared	⅔ cup	150	5	1.5	1 [P]
Baked, with skin, 2¼" – 3¼"	1 med	161	0	0	0
Baked, no skin, 2⅔" – 4¾"	1 med	145	0	0	0
Canned	½ cup	54	0	0	0
Russet, baked, with skin, 2¼" – 3¼"	1 med	168	0	0	0
Red, baked, with skin, 2¼" – 3¼"	1 med	154	0	0	0
Hash Browns, Cascadian Farms®, Organic, frozen, unprepared	1 cup	60	0	0	0
Hash Browns, Ore Ida®, frozen, unprepared	¾ cup	80	0	0	0
French Fries, Ore Ida®, Seasoned Fajita, frozen, unprepared	15 fries	160	7	1.5	na [P]
French Fries, Ore Ida®, Steak Fries, frozen, unprepared	7 fries	120	3	1	na [P]
Mashed, fresh, with milk, prepared at home	½ cup	87	1	0	na
Mashed, Alexia®, all natural, Yukon Gold Potatoes and Sea Salt, frozen	½ cup	150	6	↑4	0

Chol (mg)	Sod (mg)	Carb (g)	Fiber (g)	Sugar (g)	Prot (g)
0	35	2	1	0	0
0	4	6	2	3	1
0	0	1	0	0	0
0	368	1	1	0	0
0	⬆580	1	0	0	0
0	30	2	1	0	0
0	5	7	3	5	1
0	4	12	2	0	2
0	⬆650	22	1	3	3
0	24	37	4	2	4
0	8	34	2	3	3
0	197	12	2	0	1
0	24	37	4	2	5
0	21	34	3	2	4
0	10	14	1	0	2
0	55	18	2	0	2
0	370	22	2	0	2
0	340	17	2	1	2
0	317	18	2	2	2
20	80	20	2	1	3

Item	Serving	Cal	Total Fat (g)	Sat Fat (g)	Trans Fat (g)
Potatoes continued					
Mashed, Country Crock®, Home Style, frozen	⅔ cup	190	10	↑5	0 [P]
Mashed, dehydrated, prepared with milk, water, margarine	½ cup	122	5	2	na
Mashed, from flakes, Betty Crocker® Sour Cream and Chives, prepared	½ cup	160	7	2	1.5 [P]
Scalloped, boxed, Betty Crocker®, Prepared	½ cup	90	4	1	1 [P]
Pumpkin					
Raw	1 cup	30	0	0	0
Canned	1 cup	83	0	0	0
Radicchio					
Raw	½ cup	5	0	0	0
Radishes					
Raw, ¾" – 1"	1 med	1	0	0	0
Rutabaga					
Raw, cubes	½ cup	25	0	0	0
Sauerkraut					
Canned	½ cup	13	0	0	0
Canned, low sodium	½ cup	16	0	0	0
Scallions (green onions)					
Raw, 4⅛"	1 med	5	0	0	0
Shallots					
Raw, chopped	1 tbsp	7	0	0	0
Spinach					
Raw	1 cup	7	0	0	0
Frozen	½ cup	24	0	0	0
Canned, Popeye®	½ cup	45	0	0	0
Creamed, Bird's Eye®, frozen	½ cup	70	2.5	1	1 [P]
Sprouts					
Alfalfa, raw	¼ cup	2	0	0	0
Squash					
Acorn, baked	½ cup	57	0	0	0
Butternut, baked	½ cup	41	0	0	0

Vegetables and Vegetable Juices

Chol (mg)	Sod (mg)	Carb (g)	Fiber (g)	Sugar (g)	Prot (g)
20	450	22	2	2	3
2	180	17	1	2	2
5	↑470	21	1	3	3
0	↑630	22	0 [E]	3	3
0	1	8	1	2	1
0	↑590	20	1	8	3
0	4	1	0	0	0
0	2	0	0	0	0
0	14	6	2	4	1
0	↑469	3	2	1	1
0	219	3	2	1	1
0	2	1	0	0	0
0	1	2	0	0	0
0	24	1	1	0	1
0	58	3	2	1	3
0	200	5	3	0	0
0	↑520	9	1	4 [A]	3
0	0	0	0	0	0
0	4	15	↑5	0	1
0	4	11	na	2	1

Vegetables and Vegetable Juices | 45

Item	Serving	Cal	Total Fat (g)	Sat Fat (g)	Trans Fat (g)
Squash *continued*					
Hubbard, cooked	½ cup	51	0	0	0
Spaghetti, cooked	½ cup	21	0	0	0
Zucchini, raw, with skin	½ cup	9	0	0	0
Zucchini, cooked, with skin	½ cup	14	0	0	0
Sweet Potato					
Baked, with skin, 2" – 5"	1 med	103	0	0	0
Canned	½ cup	106	0	0	0
Candied, at home	1 med	151	0	0	0
Tomatillo					
Raw, chopped	½ cup	21	0	0	0
Tomato					
Raw, 2⅜"	1 med	22	0	0	0
Canned, Del Monte®, diced	½ cup	25	0	0	0
Canned, Muir Glen®, Organic, paste	2 tbsp	30	0	0	0
Canned, Del Monte®, with Basil, Garlic and Oregano, diced	½ cup	50	0	0	0
Canned, S&W®, with Garlic, Oregano and Basil, diced	½ cup	25	0	0	0
Canned, Hunts®, sauce	¼ cup	15	0	0	0
Canned, Del Monte®, stewed	½ cup	35	0	0	0
Cherry, raw	½ cup	13	0	0	0
Plum, raw	1	11	0	0	0
Sun-dried, in oil	¼ cup	59	4	0	0
Sun-dried, no oil	¼ cup	35	0	0	0
Juice, R.W. Knudsen® Organic Tomato	8 oz	60	0	0	0
Juice, Campbell®, original	5.5oz can	30	0	0	0
Juice, Campbell®, low sodium	8 oz	50	0	0	0
Taro					
Raw	½ cup	58	0	0	0
Turnip Greens					
Raw	½ cup	9	0	0	0

Chol (mg)	Sod (mg)	Carb (g)	Fiber (g)	Sugar (g)	Prot (g)
0	8	11	na	0	3
0	14	5	1	2	1
0	6	2	1	1	1
0	3	4	1	2	1
0	41	24	4	7	2
0	38	25	3	6	1
0	74	29	3	na	1
0	1	4	1	3	1
0	6	5	2	3	1
0	250	6	2	4	1
0	20	6	1	3	1
0	↑650	11	0	8	2
0	190	4	0	4	1
0	360	3	1	2	0
0	360	9	2	7	1
0	4	3	1	2	1
0	3	2	1	2	1
0	73	6	2	na	1
0	283	8	2	5	2
0	390	14	0	8	2
0	↑520	6	1	5	1
0	140	10	2	7	2
0	6	14	2	0	1
0	11	2	1	0	0

Vegetables and Vegetable Juices

Item	Serving	Cal	Total Fat (g)	Sat Fat (g)	Trans Fat (g)
Turnips					
Raw	1 med	34	0	0	0
Vegetable Juice					
Juice, R.W. Knudsen ® Organic Very Veggie	8 oz	50	0	0	0
Juice, R.W. Knudsen ® Organic Very Veggie, low sodium	8 oz	50	0	0	0
V8®, original	8 oz	50	0	0	0
V8®, low sodium	8 oz	50	0	0	0
V8®, Splash, Berry Blend	8 oz	70	0	0	0
Water Chestnuts					
Canned	4	14	0	0	0
Watercress					
Raw	½ cup	2	0	0	0
Yams					
Canned, S&W®, candied	½ cup	170	0	0	0

Chol (mg)	Sod (mg)	Carb (g)	Fiber (g)	Sugar (g)	Prot (g)
0	82	8	2	5	1
0	↑580	11	2	7	2
0	35	14	2	8	2
0	460	10	2	8	2
0	140	10	2	8	2
0	50	18	0	18 [HF]	0
0	2	3	1	1	0
0	7	0	0	0	0
0	360	46	4	21	2

Vegetables and Vegetable Juices

The Grain Group

The Grain Group covers many types of food including any food made from wheat, oats, rice, cornmeal, barley or other cereal grain. Breads, crackers, cereal, oatmeal, grits, pasta and rice are examples of Grain products. In this section, the Grain Group is divided into two chapters, **Bread and Cereal** and **Grains, Pasta and Rice** products.

USDA Recommendations:

Make half of your Grains Whole.

Aim for at least 3 Whole Grains a day.

KEEP IT SIMPLE

Eat 6 ounces of Grains per day— from the entire Grain Group. *USDA recommended Daily Serving is based on a 2,000 calorie diet.*

Grains and all plant foods **contain fiber.** A high-fiber diet can help lower your risk of heart disease, cancer and diabetes.

Grains **do not contain cholesterol** and are **naturally low in fat.** It is what's added to Grain products that add the fat and cholesterol like butter and full fat dairy products.

Grains are the seeds of plants.

Whole grains include the entire seed, the germ, bran and endosperm. The bran and germ of the seed contain high amounts of **fiber** and essential nutrients.

Refined grains have been milled, a process that removes the bran, germ, fiber and nutrients.

White flour and wheat flour are examples of refined grains. Refined grains are considered to be poor in nutrition.

Enriched grains are refined grains "enriched" with vitamins lost in the milling process; however, fiber and various other B vitamins are not added back.

To find Whole Grain products, look at the INGREDIENTS list. The first or predominate Ingredient should be—"Whole" grain or "Whole" wheat. See example below:

> **INGREDIENTS: WHOLE** WHEAT FLOUR, BROWN SUGAR, HONEY, MILK PROTEIN, YEAST, SOYBEAN AND/OR COTTONSEED OIL.

Breads and Cereals

Bread and Cereal products are considered part of the USDA Food Pyramid **Grain Group.** This chapter covers **Bread, Crackers, Cereal, Pancakes, Pastries** and **Waffles.**

USDA Recommendations:

Make half your Grains Whole.

KEEP IT SIMPLE

Eat 6 ounces of Grains per day— from the entire Grain Group. *USDA recommended Daily Serving is based on a 2,000 calorie diet.*

Breads and Cereals and all plant based foods (carbohydrates) **contain fiber.** Foods coded as ↑ in fiber are excellent choices.

Refined grains are typically not identified on the INGREDIENTS list or packaging as refined. If the INGREDIENTS list does not specifically state it was made with "whole" or "enriched" flour/grains—know they are refined grains.

Products identified in this chapter with a ^{W} are whole grain foods. Choose whole grains more often.

Some Bread and Cereal products are a mix of refined, whole and enriched grains. Product packaging statements such as "made with whole grains" or "contains 2 grams of whole grains" are a sign the product may not be entirely Whole Grain.

Bread and Cereal products have little to **no cholesterol.** Products containing cholesterol are usually made with a lot of butter, i.e. croissants.

Varying amounts of **fat, saturated fat** and **sodium** can be found in Bread and Cereal products and some contain unhealthy **Trans Fats** (partially hydrogenated oils). Products containing Trans Fats should be avoided. They are coded with a [P] in this chapter.

Many Bread and Cereal products are made with High Fructose Corn Syrup and can be just as high in sugar as many desserts.

Examples of Whole and Refined Grains in this chapter:

Whole Grains

Oatmeal
Whole cornmeal
Whole wheat flour

Wheat flour
White flour

Refined Grains

Grits
Enriched wheat flour

EAT SMART. Look for products labeled Whole Grain or even better 100% Whole Grain (verify this on the INGREDIENTS list). Choose Bread and Cereal products with 5 or more grams of fiber and 5 or less grams of sugar. Minimize fat and cholesterol by topping Bread and Cereal products with low fat dairy or spreads. Always read the INGREDIENTS list of products and avoid foods made with Partially Hydrogenated Oils.

Item	Serving	Cal	Total Fat (g)	Sat Fat (g)	Trans Fat (g)

BREADS

Bagels

Item	Serving	Cal	Total Fat (g)	Sat Fat (g)	Trans Fat (g)
Cinnamon raisin – 3 inch	1	156	1	0	na
Oat bran – 3 inch	1	145	1	0	na
Plain, enriched	1	190	1	0	na

Biscuits

Item	Serving	Cal	Total Fat (g)	Sat Fat (g)	Trans Fat (g)
Buttermilk or plain, commercially baked	1 med	186	8	1	na
Buttermilk, Pillsbury® refrigerated dough	1 serv	150	2	0	0 [P]
Buttermilk, Pillsbury® GRANDS, Home Style, refrigerated dough	1 serv	190	8	3	3 [P]
Buttermilk, Bisquick®, Complete, dry	1 serv	150	6	1.5	2.5 [P]
Plain, Bisquick®, Heart Smart, dry	1 serv	140	2.5	0	0
Plain, Bisquick®, original, dry	1 serv	160	5	1.5	1.5 [P]
Breadstick, plain	1 med	41	1	0	na

Cornbread

Item	Serving	Cal	Total Fat (g)	Sat Fat (g)	Trans Fat (g)
Betty Crocker®, dry mix, unprepared	1 serv	110	1	0	.5 [P]
Jiffy®, dry mix, unprepared	1 serv	150	4.5	2	0 [H,P]
Croissant, butter	1 med	231	12	↑6	na
Focaccia, Buitoni®, Italian Herb & Cheese, dry bread mix.	1 serv	110	2	.5	0 [P]
French Bread	1 med	185	1	0	na
Grain sprouted Bread, Ezeikel®, low sodium	1 slice	80	.5	0	0
Italian Bread – 4" x 2½"	1 slice	81	1	0	na
Mixed-grain Bread	1 slice	65	1	0	na
Qat Bran Bread	1 slice	71	1	0	na
Pumpernickel Bread	1 slice	65	1	0	na
Raisin Bread	1 slice	71	1	0	na
Rye Bread	1 slice	83	1	0	na
Sourdough Bread – 4" x 2½"	1 slice	185	1	0	na

Chol (mg)	Sod (mg)	Carb (g)	Fiber (g)	Sugar (g)	Prot (g)
0	184	31	1	3	6
0	289	30	2	1	6
0	368	37	2	0	7
0	↑537	25	1	2	3
0	↑570	29	1	4	4
0	↑600	24	1	4	4
0	370	21	1	1	3
0	430	27	1	3	3
0	↑490	26	1	1	3
0	66	7	0	0	1
0	210	24	1	6	2
5	340	27	1	2	7
38	424	26	2	6	5
0	390	21	0	3	3
0	416	36	2	2	8
0	0	15	3 W	0	4
0	175	15	1	0	3
0	127	12	2	3	3
0	122	12	1	2	3
0	174	12	2	0	2
0	101	14	1	0	2
0	211	15	2	1	3
0	416	36	2	2	8

Item	Serving	Cal	Total Fat (g)	Sat Fat (g)	Trans Fat (g)
White Bread					
Sara Lee®, Soft & Smooth, Classic White	1 slice	80	1	.5	0
Sara Lee®, Soft & Smooth, made with whole grain	1 slice	70	1	.5	0
Wheat Bread					
Roman Meal®, Split Top	1 slice	80	1	0	0
Whole Grain Bread					
Milton's®, Whole Grain	1 slice	90	.5	0	0
Sara Lee®, Home Style 100% Whole Wheat	1 slice	100	1.5	0	0
Sara Lee®, 100% Natural, 100% Whole Wheat with Honey	1 slice	110	1.5	0.5	0
Buns & Rolls					
Crescent Rolls, Pillsbury®, original Refrigerated	1 roll	110	6	2	1.5 [P]
Crescent Rolls, Pillsbury®, reduced fat, Refrigerated	1 roll	90	4.5	2	0 [P]
French Roll, Francisco®	1 roll	110	1.5	0	0
Potato Hamburger Buns, Aunt Hatties®	1 bun	140	2	0	0
Potato Hotdog Buns, Aunt Hatties®	1 bun	140	2	0	0
Sourdough Rolls, Francisco®	1 roll	110	1	0	0
Wheat, Sara Lee®, Wheat made with Honey, Dinner Rolls	1 roll	110	1.5	0	0
Whole Wheat, Oroweat® 100% Whole Wheat, Dinner Rolls	1 roll	130	1.5	0	0
Croutons, Rothbury Farms®, Organic, seasoned whole grain	2 tbsp	30	1	0	0
English Muffins					
Oroweat®, 100% Whole Wheat	1	130	1.5	0	0
Wonder®, Sourdough	1	130	.5	0	0
Pitas					
Low Carb, Toufayan®	1	130	2.5	0	0

Chol (mg)	Sod (mg)	Carb (g)	Fiber (g)	Sugar (g)	Prot (g)
0	140	15	1	2 [HF]	2
0	125	14	2 [E,W]	3 [HF]	3
0	150	15	1 [W,R]	3 [HF]	3
0	125	16	↑5 [W]	3	4
0	190	20	2 [W]	3 [HF]	5
0	210	21	3 [W]	4	5
0	220	11	0	2	2
0	220	12	0	2	2
0	250	21	1	1 [HF]	4
0	220	25	1	4 [HF]	4
0	250	25	1	4 [HF]	5
0	180	21	1	1 [HF]	4
0	200	20	1 [E,W]	3 [HF]	4
0	260	23	4 [W]	4 [HF]	6
0	65	4	1 [W]	0	1
0	240	26	4 [W]	6	6
0	220	26	1	2 [HF]	5
0	↑580	16	↑9 [W]	0	11

The Grain Group | 57

Item	Serving	Cal	Total Fat (g)	Sat Fat (g)	Trans Fat (g)
Pitas continued					
White – 6½"	1	165	1	0	na
Whole Grain, Thomas® Sahara®	1	140	1.5	0	0
Whole Wheat – 6½"	1	170	2	0	na
Stuffing, Kraft® Stove Top, chicken stuffing mix, dry, prepared	½ cup	160	7	1.5	1.5 P
Tortillas					
Corn, Tortillas	1	52	1	0	na
Flour Tortillas, Mission®, 7" – 96% fat Free	1	130	1.5	0	.5 H,P
Whole Wheat, Tortillas, Mission® 7"	1	130	2	0	0 H,P
Whole Wheat, Tortillas, La Tortillas®, 7"	1	50	2	0	0
Whole Wheat, Tortillas, La Tortillas®, 8"	1	80	3	0	0
Crackers					
All Bran, Kellogg®, Multi-Gain Crackers	18	130	6	1	0
Buttery Baked Crackers, Back to Nature®, Classic Rounds	5	70	2	0	0
Cheese, Back to Nature®, Crispy Cheddars	24	140	5	.5	0
Cheez-It®, original	27	160	8	2	0 P
Club®, original	4	70	3	1	0 P
Club®, reduced fat	5	70	2.5	.5	0 P
Milton's®, Multi-Grain, Baked Crackers	14	140	6	0	0
Milton's®, Whole Wheat, Baked Crackers	14	130	6	0	0
Pepperidge Farm®, Goldfish, Baked Crackers	55	150	6	.5	0
Pepperidge Farm®, Hearty Wheat	3	80	0	0	0
Ritz®, original	5	80	4	1	0 P
Ritz®, original, reduced fat	5	70	2	0	0 P
Saltine, Premium®, original – 16oz pkg.	5	60	1.5	0	0 P

Chol (mg)	Sod (mg)	Carb (g)	Fiber (g)	Sugar (g)	Prot (g)
0	322	33	1	0	5
0	310	27	4 W	2 HF	6
0	340	35	↑5	1	6
0	↑510	21	1	2 HF	3
0	11	11	2	0	1
0	330	26	3	2	4
0	340	25	3 W	3	4
0	180	11	↑8 W	0	5
0	300	19	↑14 W	1	8
0	270	19	↑5 W	4	2
0	150	11	0	1	1
0	320	20	1	0	3
0	250	18	1	1	4
0	150	9	1	1 HF	1
0	190	12	1	2 HF	1
0	240	18	1 E,W	2	3
0	260	18	1 E,W	2	3
0	230	20	1 W	1	3
0	100	10	1 E,W	2	2
0	135	10	0	1 HF	1
0	150	11	0	1 HF	1
0	190	11	0	0 HF	1

The Grain Group

Item	Serving	Cal	Total Fat (g)	Sat Fat (g)	Trans Fat (g)
Crackers continued					
Saltine, Premium®, low sodium – 16oz pkg.	5	60	1.5	0	0 [P]
Saltine, Premium®, Multi Grain – 16oz. pkg.	5	60	1.5	0	0 [P]
Sociables, Nabisco®	5	70	3.5	.5	0 [P]
Triscuit®, original	7	120	4.5	.5	0
Triscuit®, reduced fat	7	120	3	0	0
Wasa®, Fibre	1	32	1	0	0
Wasa®, Sesame, Crisp bread	1	60	1	0	0
Wheat Thins®, original	16	150	6	1	0
Wheat Thins®, original, reduced fat	16	130	4	.5	0
Wheat Thins®, multi-grain chips	12	120	4	.5	0
Wheat Crackers, Back to Nature®, Crispy Wheat Baked Crackers	17	130	4	0	0
Wheat Crackers, Wheatsworth®, stone ground wheat	5	80	3.5	1	0 [H, P]
Whole Grain, Back to Nature®, Harvest 100% Whole Grain Baked Crackers	6	120	4.5	0	0
Zesta®, original	5	60	1.5	0	0

CEREALS

Cereal: ready to eat, dry					
All-Bran, Kellogg®, Complete, Wheat Flakes	¾ cup	90	.5	0	0
All-Bran, Kellogg®, Extra Fiber	½ cup	50	1	0	0
All-Bran, Kellogg®, original	½ cup	81	2	0	0
CAP'N Crunch, Quaker®, original	¾ cup	110	1.5	1	0
CAP'N Crunch, Quaker®, Crunch Berries	¾ cup	100	1.5	1	0 [P]
Cascadian Farms, Honeynut O's, General Mills®, Organic	1 cup	120	1.5	0	0

Chol (mg)	Sod (mg)	Carb (g)	Fiber (g)	Sugar (g)	Prot (g)
0	25	11	0	0	1
0	170	10	0 E,W	0	1
0	140	9	0 E,W	1 HF	1
0	180	19	3 W	0	3
0	160	21	3 W	0	3
0	0	5	2.5 W	0	1.5
0	70	9	1	0	2
0	260	21	1 E,W	4 HF	2
0	260	21	1 E,W	4 HF	2
0	290	20	1 E,W	3 HF	2
0	290	22	1	4	3
0	180	10	1 E,W	1	2
0	180	19	3 W	0	3
0	200	11	1 E	0	1

0	210	23	↑5 W	5 HF	3
0	120	20	↑13	0 A	3
0	75	23	↑9	5 HF	4
0	200	23	1	12	1
0	180	22	1	12	1
0	250	24	2 W	8	3

The Grain Group

Item	Serving	Cal	Total Fat (g)	Sat Fat (g)	Trans Fat (g)
Cereal: ready to eat, dry *continued*					
Cascadian Farms, Purely O's, General Mills®, Organic	1 cup	110	2	.5	0
Chex, Multi-Bran, General Mills®	1 cup	180	1	0	0
Cheerios, General Mills®, plain	1 cup	110	2	0	0
Cheerios, General Mills®, Honeynut	¾ cup	110	1.5	0	0
Cocoa Puffs, General Mills®	1 cup	120	2	0	0
Corn Flakes, Kellogg®	1 cup	101	0	0	0
Ezekiel 4:9®, Golden Flax	½ cup	180	2.5	0	0
Fiber One, General Mills®	½ cup	60	1	0	0
Frosted Flakes, Kellogg®	¾ cup	114	0	0	0
Frosted Mini-Wheats, Kellogg®	1 cup	175	1	0	0
Frosted Mini-Wheats, Kellogg®, Organic	24	190	1	0	0
Fruit Loops, Kellogg®	1 cup	118	1	0	.5 [P]
Grape Nuts, Kraft POST®	½ cup	208	1	0	0
Honey Bunches of Oats, Kraft POST®, Honey roasted	½ cup	120	1.5	0	0
Honeycomb, Kraft POST®	1½ cups	120	1	0	0
Kashi, Organic Promise®, Autumn Wheat	1 cup	190	1	0	0
Kashi, Organic Promise®, Cinnamon Harvest	1 cup	190	1	0	0
Life, Quaker®, original	¾ cup	120	1.5	0	0
Lucky Charms, General Mills®	1 cup	120	1	0	0
Raisin Bran, Kellogg®	1 cup	195	2	0	0
Raisin Bran, Kellogg®, Organic	1 cup	190	1	0	0
Rice Krispies, Kellogg®	1 cup	108	0	0	0
Rice Krispies, Kellogg®, Organic	1¼ cup	120	0	0	0
Smart Start, Kellogg®, original	1 cup	230	3	0	0

Chol (mg)	Sod (mg)	Carb (g)	Fiber (g)	Sugar (g)	Prot (g)
0	280	22	3 W	1	3
0	342	46	↑7 W	11	4
0	210	23	3 W	1	3
0	190	22	2 W	9	3
0	160	26	1.5 W	14	1
0	202	24	1	3 HF	2
0	190	37	↑6 W	0	8
0	105	25	↑14 W	0	2
0	148	28	1	12 HF	1
0	5	41	↑5 W	10 HF	5
0	0	44	↑5 W	11	4
0	150	26	1	12	2
0	354	47	↑5 W	7	6
0	150	25	2 W	6	2
0	170	28	3 W	10	2
0	0	45	↑6 W	7	5
0	0	44	↑5 W	9	4
0	160	25	2 W	6	3
0	200	25	1 W	13	3
0	362	47	↑7 W	20 HF	5
0	380	46	↑8 W	16	5
0	266	24	0	3 HF	2
0	320	29	0	3	2
0	140	46	↑5	17 HF	7

The Grain Group

Item	Serving	Cal	Total Fat (g)	Sat Fat (g)	Trans Fat (g)
Cereal: ready to eat, dry *continued*					
Special K, Kellogg®	1 cup	117	0	0	0
Special K, Kellogg®, low carb	¾ cup	101	3	1	0
Total Raisin Bran, General Mills®	1 cup	170	1	0	0
Trix, General Mills®	1 cup	120	1.5	0	0
Wheaties, General Mills®	1 cup	110	1	0	0
Cereal: hot, cooked					
Corn Grits, yellow, cooked with water, no salt	1 cup	143	0	0	0
Corn Grits, Quaker®, Quick Grits, plain, cooked with water	1 pkt	93	0	0	0
Corn Grits, Quaker®, Country Bacon, instant, cooked with water	1 pkt	97	0	0	0
Cream of Rice®, original, instant, Cooked with water, no salt	1 cup	127	0	0	0
Cream of Wheat®, original, instant, Cooked with water, no salt	1 cup	131	1	0	0
Malt-O-Meal®, Chocolate, instant, cooked with water, no salt	1 serv	118	0	0	0
Malt-O-Meal®, original, cooked with water, no salt	1 serv	113	0	0	0
Oatmeal, Quaker®, Organic, instant, prepared with water	1 pkt	100	2	0	0
Oatmeal, Quaker®, Apple Crisp, instant, prepared with water	1 pkt	150	2	0	0 [P]
Oatmeal, Quaker®, Cinnamon Spice, instant, made with water	1 pkt	177	2	0	0
Oatmeal, Quaker®, Old Fashion, 100% whole grain dry oats	½ cup	150	3	.5	0
Oatmeal, Quaker®, Steel Cut Oats, 100% whole grain dry oats	¼ cup	150	2.5	.5	0

Chol (mg)	Sod (mg)	Carb (g)	Fiber (g)	Sugar (g)	Prot (g)
0	244	22	1	4 HF	7
0	110	14	↑5 W	2 HF	10
0	240	42	↑5 W	19	3
0	190	26	1 W	13 HF	1
0	210	24	3 W	4	3
0	5	31	1	0	3
0	288	21	1	0	2
0	413	21	1	0	3
0	2	28	0	0	2
0	8	28	1	0	4
0	8	25	1	8	3
0	8	23	1	0	4
0	0	19	3 W	0	4
0	220	31	3 W	13	3
0	249	36	3 W	16	4
0	0	27	4 W	1	5
0	0	27	4 W	1	5

The Grain Group | 65

Item	Serving	Cal	Total Fat (g)	Sat Fat (g)	Trans Fat (g)

PANCAKES, PASTRIES and WAFFLES

Pancakes

Item	Serving	Cal	Total Fat (g)	Sat Fat (g)	Trans Fat (g)
Pancake, Buttermilk, Aunt Jemima®, Complete dry mix 1/3 cup, prepared	3 cakes	160	2	.5	0 P
Pancake, Buttermilk, Hungry Jack®, Complete dry mix 1/3 cup, prepared	3 cakes	150	1.5	0	0 P
Pancake, Buttermilk, Krusteaz®, Complete dry mix 1/2 cup dry, prepared	3 cakes	210	2	.5	.5 P
Pancake, Multi-Grain Buttermilk, Hodgson Mill®, with flax seed & soy 1/3 cup dry mix, prepared	2 cakes	150	2	0	0
Pancake, Fast food, with syrup and butter	2 cakes	520	↑14	↑6	na

Pastries

Item	Serving	Cal	Total Fat (g)	Sat Fat (g)	Trans Fat (g)
Apple, Toaster Pops, Amy's®	1	150	3.5	0	0
Cheese, Danish – 4¼"	1	266	↑16	↑5	0 P
Cinnamon roll with frosting – 4"	1	217	8	2	0 P
Fruit, Danish – 4¼"	1	263	↑13	3	0 P
Poptarts®, Blueberry, Kellogg's®	1	210	6	2	0 H
Poptarts®, Frosted Brown Sugar Cinnamon, Kellogg's®	1	210	7	2.5	0 H
Poptarts®, Frosted Brown Sugar Cinnamon, Kellogg's®, low fat	1	190	3	1	0 H
Poptarts®, Frosted Cherry, Kellogg's®	1	200	5	2.5	0 H, P
Poptarts®, Frosted Chocolate Fudge, Kellogg's®	1	200	5	1.5	0 H, P
Toaster Strudel®, Apple, Pillsbury®	1	190	9	↑3.5	1 P
Toaster Strudel®, Blueberry, Pillsbury®	1	190	9	↑3.5	1 P
Toaster Strudel®, Cherry, Pillsbury®	1	190	8	↑3.5	1 P

Chol (mg)	Sod (mg)	Carb (g)	Fiber (g)	Sugar (g)	Prot (g)
0	460	31	1	6	5
5	↑550	31	1	7	4
5	↑560	42	1	6	6
0	321	31	↑5 W	2	10
↑58	↑1104	↑91	na	na	8
0	110	26	1	8	4
11	320	26	1	5	6
0	↑499	34	0	na	3
81	251	34	1	20	4
0	180	37	1	16 HF	2
0	170	34	1	16 HF	2
0	210	38	1	19 HF	2
0	160	38	1	16 HF	2
0	210	37	1	20 HF	3
5	190	26	1	9 HF	3
5	190	26	1	9 HF	3
5	190	25	1	9 HF	3

The Grain Group | 67

Item	Serving	Cal	Total Fat (g)	Sat Fat (g)	Trans Fat (g)
Waffles					
Eggo®, Nutri-Grain, Whole Wheat, low fat, frozen	1	71	1	0	0
Eggo® Home Style, frozen	1	180	6	2	0
Van's® Organic, Blueberry, frozen	2	240	10	1.5	0
Van's® Organic, Flax, frozen	2	230	11	1.5	0
Van's® Organic, Original, frozen	2	190	4.5	0	0

Chol (mg)	Sod (mg)	Carb (g)	Fiber (g)	Sugar (g)	Prot (g)
0	215	14	1 [E,W]	2	2
20	440	27	1	2	5
0	320	29	4 [W]	2	5
0	230	26	↑6 [W]	4	6
0	230	30	↑6 [W]	4	6

The Grain Group

Grains, Pasta and Rice

Grains, Pasta and **Rice** is part of the USDA Food Pyramid **Grain Group**.

USDA Recommendations:

Make half your Grains Whole.

KEEP IT SIMPLE

Eat 6 ounces of Grains per day— from the entire Grain Group. *USDA recommended Daily Serving is based on a 2,000 calorie diet.*

Grains, Pasta and Rice and all plant based foods (carbohydrates) **contain fiber.** Foods coded as ⬆ in fiber are excellent choices.

Grains, Pasta and Rice are plant derived products and **do not contain cholesterol,** unless they're made with eggs, i.e. egg noodles.

Grains, Pasta and Rice are naturally **low in sodium, fat, saturated fat** and sugar.

It's what's added to Grains, Pasta and Rice that adds the fat and cholesterol. Butter, margarine, eggs, cheese and creamy sauces instantly add fat, saturated fat, cholesterol and even Trans Fats to Grain products.

Flavored Pasta and Rice dishes may contain more than 50% of the recommended Daily Value for **sodium.** These products may also contain High Fructose Corn Syrup and **Trans Fats** (partially hydrogenated oils). Food containing Partially Hydrogenated Oils are coded with a ᴾ in the Trans Fat column of this chapter.

Products identified in this chapter with a ^W are whole grain foods. Choose whole grains more often.

Examples of Whole and Refined Grains in this chapter:

Whole Grains

Barley
Brown Rice
Bulgur
Wild Rice

Refined Grains

Pearled barley
White Rice
Couscous

EAT SMART. To reduce fat top Pasta and Rice with tomato based sauces, low fat cheese or low fat cream sauces. Trim down sodium by choosing plain products over flavored products. Season plain products with garlic and onions and/or your favorite fresh or dried herbs. Always read the INGREDIENTS list and steer clear of products containing "partially hydrogenated" oils.

Item	Serving	Cal	Total Fat (g)	Sat Fat (g)	Trans Fat (g)
GRAINS					
Barley, pearled, cooked	½ cup	97	0	0	0
Bulgur Wheat, dry	½ cup	239	1	0	0
Cornmeal, whole grain, yellow	½ cup	221	2	0	0
Hominy, yellow	½ cup	58	1	0	0
Kasha (Buckwheat groats), cooked	½ cup	77	1	0	0
Masa (corn flour)	½ cup	208	2	0	0
Millet, cooked	½ cup	104	1	0	0
Oat Bran, cooked	½ cup	44	1	0	0
Quinoa	½ cup	318	5	1	0
Tabbouleh, Fantastic®, dry, prepared	⅓ cup	150	1	0	0
Wheat Germ, Hodgson Mills®, un-toasted	2 tbsp	55	1	0	0
Wheat Germ, Quaker® Kretschmer, toasted	2 tbsp	50	0	0	0
Couscous					
Cooked	½ cup	88	0	0	0
Far East®, Mediterranean Curry, dry, prepared	1 cup	220	4	.5	0
Far East®, Original, dry, prepared	1 cup	230	2	0	0
Hodgson Mill's®, Whole Grain, dry	⅓ cup	230	2	0	0
Noodles *(Note: 2 oz. dry = 1 cup cooked)*					
Egg, cooked	1 cup	221	3	1	0
Japanese, Somen, cooked	1 cup	231	0	0	0
Rice, cooked	1 cup	192	0	0	0
Rice noodles, De Boles®, Spaghetti style, dry	¼ pkg	210	.5	0	0

PASTA

Item	Serving	Cal	Total Fat (g)	Sat Fat (g)	Trans Fat (g)
Angel Hair					
American Beauty®, dry	2 oz	210	1	0	0
De Boles®, Tomato and Basil, Organic, dry	2 oz	210	1	0	0
Naturally Preferred®, Organic, dry	2 oz	210	1	0	0

Chol (mg)	Sod (mg)	Carb (g)	Fiber (g)	Sugar (g)	Prot (g)
0	2	22	3	0	2
0	12	53	↑13 W	0	9
0	21	47	↑5 W	0	5
0	168	11	2	0	1
0	3	17	2	1	3
0	3	43	na	na	5
0	2	21	1 W	0	3
0	1	13	3	0	4
0	18	↑59	↑5	0	11
0	↑550	33	↑6	1	5
0	0	7	4	0	4
0	0	6	2	2	4
0	4	18	1	0	3
0	↑550	40	3	2	8
0	5	46	2	1	8
0	↑630	50	↑6 W	1	10
46	8	40	2	1	7
0	283	48	na	na	7
0	33	44	2	na	2
0	15	46	1	0	4

0	0	42	2	2	1
0	5	43	2	1	7
0	0	42	2	3	7

The Grain Group

Item	Serving	Cal	Total Fat (g)	Sat Fat (g)	Trans Fat (g)
Angel Hair *continued*					
De Boles®, Tomato and Basil, Organic, dry	2 oz	210	1	0	0
Corn					
Corn, cooked	1 cup	176	1	0	0
De Boles®, Elbow style, Wheat free, dry	⅙ pkg	200	2	0	0
Fettuccini					
American Beauty®, dry	2 oz	210	1	0	0
De Boles®, Organic, dry	2 oz	210	1	0	0
De Boles®, Spinach, Organic, dry	2 oz	210	1	0	0
Lasagna					
Barilla®, dry	2 oz	180	1	0	0
De Boles®, Organic, dry	2.5 oz	260	1	0	0
Manicotti					
American Beauty®, dry	2 oz	210	1	0	0
Penne					
De Boles®, Whole Wheat, Organic, dry	2 oz	210	1.5	0	0
Heartland®, Organic, cooked	¾ cup	210	1	0	0
Shells, American Beauty®, Jumbo, dry	7	210	0	0	0
Spaghetti					
De Boles®, Organic, dry	2 oz	210	1	0	0
De Boles®, Whole Wheat, Organic, dry	2 oz	210	1	0	0
Ezekiel 4:9®, Sprouted Whole Grain, dry	2 oz	210	2	.5	0
Healthy Harvest®, Whole Wheat Blend, thin spaghetti, dry	2 oz	210	1.5	0	0
Pasta, Dishes					
Hamburger Helper®, Beef Pasta, prepared	1 cup	270	11	↑4.5	.5 ᴾ
Hamburger Helper®, Chicken, prepared	1 cup	300	12	↑3.5	1.5 ᴾ
Hamburger Helper®, Spaghetti, prepared	1 cup	280	11	↑4	.5 ᴾ
Knorr-Lipton®, Pasta Sides®, Alfredo, dry mix, unprepared	⅔ cup	240	4.5	2.5	0

Chol (mg)	Sod (mg)	Carb (g)	Fiber (g)	Sugar (g)	Prot (g)
0	5	43	2	1	7
0	0	39	↑7	na	4
0	15	43	↑5	0	4
0	0	42	2	2	7
0	5	43	1	2	7
0	20	43	3	1	7
0	0	38	2	1	6
0	5	54	1	2	9
0	0	24	2	2	7
0	10	42	↑5 [W]	2	7
0	0	41	2	2	7
0	0	42	2	2	7
0	5	43	1	2	7
0	10	42	↑5 [W]	2	7
0	10	39	↑7 [W]	0	9
0	0	42	↑3 [E,W]	2	7
55	↑810	24	1	3	20
55	↑770	26	1	5	24
55	↑870	26	1	5	20
10	↑810	40	1	3	8

The Grain Group | 75

Item	Serving	Cal	Total Fat (g)	Sat Fat (g)	Trans Fat (g)
Pasta, Dishes *continued*					
Knorr-Lipton®, Pasta Sides®, Butter & Herb, dry mix, unprepared	⅔ cup	240	3.5	1.5	0
Lasagna					
Cheese, Lean Cuisine®, Five Cheese, frozen entrée	1 serv	320	8	↑3.5	0
Cheese, Michael Angelo's®, Four Cheese, frozen entree	1 cup	400	↑22	↑12	0
Meat, Marie Calendars®, frozen entrée	1 cup	240	8	↑4	0
Meat, Stouffer®, with meat and sauce, frozen entrée	1 serv	249	8	↑4	na
Macaroni & Cheese					
Amy's®, frozen entrée	1 serv	410	↑16	↑10	0
Banquet®, frozen entrée	1 serv	390	11	↑6	0
Country Crock®, frozen	1 cup	370	↑17	↑8	.5 [P]
Kraft®, dry mix, prepared "classic"	1 cup	380	↑15	↑4	3
Kraft®, dry mix, prepared "light"	1 cup	290	5	3	0
Lean Cuisine®, frozen entrée	1 serv	290	7	↑4	0
Marie Calendar®, frozen entrée	1 cup	350	↑15	↑10	0
Stouffers®, frozen	1 cup	350	17	↑7	0 [H, P]
Velveeta, dry mix, prepared	1 cup	360	12	↑4	0
Spaghetti					
Campbell's®, Spaghetti O's, original, canned, entrée	1 cup	180	1	.5	0
Campbell's® Spaghetti O's, with meat balls, canned, entrée	1 cup	240	8	↑3.5	.5
Chef Boyardee®, Spaghetti and Meatballs, canned, entrée	1 cup	270	10	↑4.5	0
Healthy Choice, frozen entrée	1 meal	220	3.5	1	0
Lean Cuisine®, Spaghetti with Meat Sauce, frozen entree	1 serv	284	4	1	.5

Chol (mg)	Sod (mg)	Carb (g)	Fiber (g)	Sugar (g)	Prot (g)
5	↑730	44	1	4	7
25	↑690	44	4	11	19
↑60	↑550	28	↑5	0	24
20	↑870	28	4	6	13
28	↑671	27	2	5	17
40	↑590	47	3	6	16
20	↑1100	↑58	3	6	15
40	↑940	40	1	6	14
10	↑740	49	1	7	9
10	↑600	49	1	7	9
20	↑620	41	2	8	15
45	↑1130	36	3	9	16
25	↑920	34	2	2	15
20	↑940	49	2	4	13
5	↑850	37	3	13 [HF]	6
15	↑890	32	4	10 [HF]	11
20	↑900	32	2	8 [HF]	11
10	↑510	36	5	7	10
13	↑548	49	↑5	8	14

The Grain Group

Item	Serving	Cal	Total Fat (g)	Sat Fat (g)	Trans Fat (g)
Ravioli					
Amy's®, Bowls, Cheese Ravioli, frozen	1 serv	380	12	↑4.5	0
Chef Boyardee®, Tomato and Meat Sauce, canned entrée	1 cup	240	8	3	0
Lean Cuisine®, Cheese, frozen entrée	1 serv	240	6	↑3.5	0
Tortellini					
Amy's®, Bowls, Pesto Tortellini, frozen	1 serv	430	↑19	↑8	0
Italian Village®, Cheese, frozen	1 cup	250	3	1	0

RICE

Item	Serving	Cal	Total Fat (g)	Sat Fat (g)	Trans Fat (g)
Basmati, white, Lundberg®, Long grain, dry	¼ cup	180	.5	0	0
Brown, medium grain, cooked	½ cup	109	1	0	0
Brown, Uncle Ben's®, instant, cooked	1 cup	170	1.5	0	0
Brown, Minute®, instant, dry, cooked	1 cup	170	1.5	0	0
White, medium grain, cooked	½ cup	121	0	0	0
White, Minute®, instant, dry, cooked	1 cup	200	0	0	0
White, Uncle Ben's, instant, cooked	1 cup	190	.5	0	0
Wild, cooked	½ cup	83	0	0	0
Rice, Dishes					
Knorr-Lipton®, Chicken & Broccoli, Rice Sides®, Whole Grain, dry, unprepared	⅔ cup	270	3	na	na
Rice A Roni®, Chicken & Mushroom, dry, prepared	1 cup	350	↑13	3	2 [P]
Rice A Roni®, Red Beans & Rice, dry, prepared	1 cup	290	7	1.5	1
Tai Pei®, Chicken Fried Rice, frozen	1 serv	630	↑19	2	.5 [P]
Zatarian's®, Dirty Rice with Pork	1 pkg	360	12	↑4	0

Pasta and Rice

Chol (mg)	Sod (mg)	Carb (g)	Fiber (g)	Sugar (g)	Prot (g)
25	↑680	55	4	7	14
15	↑900	35	3	5 HF	8
40	↑600	36	3	10	11
40	↑640	45	3	5	20
20	410	46	2	2	10

0	0	41	0	0	4
0	1	23	2 W	0	2
0	0	25	2 W	0	5
0	19	34	2 W	0	4
0	0	27	0	0	2
0	5	45	1	0	4
0	15	43	1	0	3
0	2	18	2 W	1	3
5	↑830	45	3 W	2	7
5	↑1430	51	2	3	8
0	↑1170	51	↑5	3	8
25	↑2160	na	↑7	15	21
15	↑1430	52	2	0	9

The Grain Group

Item	Serving	Cal	Total Fat (g)	Sat Fat (g)	Trans Fat (g)
Rice, Flavored					
Knorr-Lipton®, Beef Flavor, dry, unprepared	½ cup	240	3	3	na
Knorr-Lipton®, Chicken Flavor, dry, unprepared	½ cup	230	2	.5	na
Knorr-Lipton®, Herb & Butter, dry, unprepared	½ cup	250	4.5	2.5	0
Knorr-Lipton®, Rice Pilaf, dry, prepared	½ cup	220	2	0	na
Rice A Roni®, Beef Flavor, dry, prepared	1 cup	310	9	1.5	1.5
Rice A Roni®, Chicken Flavor, dry, prepared	1 cup	310	9	1.5	1.5
Rice A Roni®, Chicken Flavor, lower sodium, dry, prepared	1 cup	270	5	1	.5
Rice A Roni®, Rice Pilaf, dry, prepared	1 cup	310	9	1.5	1.5
Uncle Ben's®, Parmesan & Butter, dry, unprepared	2 oz	200	1	0	0
Uncle Ben's®, Oriental Fried Rice, dry, unprepared	2 oz	200	1	0	0

Chol (mg)	Sod (mg)	Carb (g)	Fiber (g)	Sugar (g)	Prot (g)
0	↑930	48	1	1	6
5	↑810	46	1	2	6
10	↑850	46	1	1	6
0	↑880	46	1	1	6
0	↑1110	51	2	3	7
0	↑1160	51	2	2	7
0	↑730	51	2	1	7
0	↑1170	51	2	1	7
0	↑860	44	1	0	5
0	↑580	42	1	1	6

The Meat and Bean Group

Foods made from meat, dry beans, peas (legumes), poultry, fish, nuts, seeds and eggs are considered part of the USDA Food Pyramid Meat and Bean Group. The Meat and Bean Group encompasses many types of foods, for that reason this section is divided into the following seven chapters:

Dry Beans, Peas and Tofu (legumes)

Nuts, Nut Butters and Seeds

Beef, Pork and Lamb

Poultry—Chicken, Duck, Goose and Turkey

Lunch Meats, Sausage and Franks

Fish and Shellfish

Eggs

USDA Recommendations:

Go lean on protein.

Vary your choices with more fish, beans, peas (legumes), nuts and seeds.

KEEP IT SIMPLE

Eat a total of 5.5 ounces per day— from the entire Meat and Bean Group. *USDA recommended Daily Serving is based on a 2,000 calorie diet.*

Dry beans and peas (legumes), nuts and seeds are plant foods (carbohydrates) within the Meat and Bean Group and are good sources of protein, **fiber** and plant nutrients.

Meat is a good source of protein, niacin, vitamins B6 and B12, iron, phosphorus, and zinc.

Fat, saturated fat and **cholesterol** are present in meat, poultry, fish and all other animal derived products, such as eggs, and dairy products. The amount varies depending on the product.

Please note, NUTRITION FACTS labeling for fresh meat, poultry and fish is optional. Most are not labeled. Compare NUTRITION FACTS in this guide to make better choices. You may be surprised just how much fat you can eliminate by choosing a different cut or grade of meat. Understanding the differences will help you make smarter/healthier choices at home or when dining out.

Dry Beans, Peas and Tofu

Dry Beans, Peas (legumes) and **Tofu** are considered part of the USDA Food Pyramid Meat and Bean Group.

USDA Recommendations:

Go lean on protein.

KEEP IT SIMPLE

Eat a total of 5.5 ounces per day— from the entire Meat and Bean Group. *USDA recommended Daily Serving is based on a 2,000 calorie diet.*

Dry Beans and Peas are an excellent source of **fiber** and protein. Most are ↑ in fiber.

Dry Beans and Peas **do not contain cholesterol** and are **naturally low in fat, saturated fat** and **sodium.**

Canned or processed beans or peas tend to be ↑ **in sodium** and may contain added sugars, **fat, saturated fat** or **Trans Fats.**

Go to Refried Beans in this chapter. Find "Traditional" Refried Beans and notice, two out of three of the canned beans contain Trans Fats (these products are coded with a [P]) including the "no fat" variety. In this case, going with the "original" variety of Traditional Refried Beans is best; they are still low in fat and they contain less sodium than the other two products.

Canned or processed beans or peas made with meats (chili or pork & beans) contain **cholesterol.**

Dry Beans, Peas and Tofu

EAT SMART. To reduce fat and sodium, home prepare Dry Bean and Peas, limit the use fat and season with herbs instead of salt. For canned beans or peas, compare the sodium content found on the NUTRITION FACTS Label with other like products, including products labeled as "low" or "less" sodium, and reduce sodium by 100mg to 500mg per serving.

Item	Serving	Cal	Total Fat (g)	Sat Fat (g)	Trans Fat (g)
DRY BEANS, PEAS and TOFU					
Baked Beans					
Plain, Bush®, Original	½ cup	140	1	0	0
Bacon & Brown Sugar, VanCamp's®, Original	½ cup	140	1	0	0
Vegetarian, Bush®	½ cup	130	0	0	0
with beef, canned	½ cup	161	5	2	na
with pork, canned	½ cup	134	2	1	na
with franks, canned	½ cup	184	9	3	na
Home, prepared	½ cup	191	7	2	0
Bean Dip					
Black Bean, Bearitos®, fat free, Vegetarian	2 tbsp	30	0	0	0
Traditional, Fritos®	2 tbsp	40	1	0	0 [P]
Black Beans					
Canned, Bush®	½ cup	100	1	0	0
Canned, Ranch Style Brand®	½ cup	100	1	0	0
Dry beans, prepared, no salt	½ cup	114	0	0	0
Black-eyed peas					
Canned, Bush®	½ cup	100	0	0	0
Cannellini					
Canned, Bush®	½ cup	90	0	0	0
Chickpeas (garbanzo)					
Canned, Westbrae Natural®, Organic Garbanzo beans	½ cup	110	2	0	0
Dry Chickpeas, prepared, no salt	½ cup	134	2	0	0
Chili					
Chili and Beans					
Hormel®, with beans, canned entrée	1 serv	270	7	3	0
Hormel®, with beans, less sodium, canned entrée	1 serv	340	↑17	↑7	0
Stagg®, Country Style, canned chili and beans	1 serv	319	↑16	↑7	0
Stagg®, Ranch House, canned chili and beans	1 serv	284	9	3	0

Chol (mg)	Sod (mg)	Carb (g)	Fiber (g)	Sugar (g)	Prot (g)
0	↑550	29	↑5	12	6
0	↑540	30	↑6	12	7
0	↑550	29	↑5	12	6
29	↑632	22	na	na	8
9	↑524	25	↑7	na	7
8	↑557	20	↑9	8	9
6	↑534	27	↑7	na	7
0	170	6	1	0	2
0	170	5	1	0	2
0	460	20	↑7	1	7
0	420	19	↑5	1	6
0	1	20	↑7	na	8
0	410	19	4	0	5
0	270	19	↑6	0	7
0	140	18	↑5	3	6
0	6	22	↑6	4	7
30	↑1200	34	↑7	5	16
60	↑900	30	↑9	3	18
40	↑1131	29	↑6	6	15
47	↑813	32	↑9	6	19

The Meat and Bean Group

Item	Serving	Cal	Total Fat (g)	Sat Fat (g)	Trans Fat (g)
Chili *continued*					
No Beans					
Hormel®, canned entrée	1 serv	210	9	3	0
Turkey					
Hormel®, with beans, canned entrée	1 serv	200	3	1	0
Vegetarian					
Hormel®, canned entrée	1 serv	205	1	0	0
Falafel					
Home, prepared	1 patty	57	3	0	0
Dry, Fantastic®, prepared	¼ cup	130	2	0	0
Fava (Broadbeans)					
Raw, pods	½ cup	55	0	0	0
Beans, canned	½ cup	91	0	0	0
Great Northern Beans					
Canned	½ cup	149	1	0	0
Dry, prepared, no salt	½ cup	104	0	0	0
Hummus					
Hummus, Fantastic®, dry mix, prepared	2 tbsp	80	3.5	0	0
Hummus, Athenos®, refrigerated	2 tbsp	50	3	0	0
Kidney Beans					
Canned	½ cup	109	0	0	0
Dry, prepared, no salt	½ cup	112	0	0	0
Lentils					
Dry, prepared, no salt	½ cup	115	0	0	0
Lima Beans					
Canned	½ cup	95	0	0	0
Dry, large beans, prepared, no salt	½ cup	108	0	0	0
Navy Beans					
Canned	½ cup	148	1	0	0
Dry beans, prepared, no salt	½ cup	127	1	0	0
Peas, Split					
Dry, prepared, no salt	½ cup	116	0	0	0

Chol (mg)	Sod (mg)	Carb (g)	Fiber (g)	Sugar (g)	Prot (g)
40	↑970	17	3	3	16
45	↑1200	26	↑5	6	17
0	↑778	38	↑10	6	12
0	50	5	na	na	2
0	350	21	↑6	3	7
0	16	11	na	na	5
0	↑580	16	↑5	na	7
0	5	28	↑6	na	10
0	2	19	↑6	na	7
0	270	11	1	0	3
0	160	5	1	1	1
0	436	20	↑8	0	7
0	2	20	↑7	0	8
0	2	20	↑8	2	9
0	405	18	↑6	na	6
0	2	20	↑7	3	7
0	↑587	27	↑7	0	10
0	0	24	↑10	0	7
0	2	21	↑8	3	8

The Meat and Bean Group | 89

Item	Serving	Cal	Total Fat (g)	Sat Fat (g)	Trans Fat (g)
Pinto Beans					
Canned	½ cup	103	1	0	0
Dry beans, prepared, no salt	½ cup	122	1	0	0
Pork and Beans					
Canned, Campbell®	½ cup	140	1.5	.5	0
Canned, VanCamp's®	½ cup	110	1	0	0
Shellie Beans					
Canned	½ cup	37	0	0	0
Soybeans, Green					
Dry, prepared, no salt	½ cup	127	6	1	0
Raw	½ cup	188	9	1	0
Ranch Style Beans					
Canned, Ranch Style® brand	½ cup	130	3	1	0 [P]
Refried Beans					
Traditional					
Fantastic®, All Natural, dry mix, prepared	¼ cup	130	2	0	0
Old El Paso®, canned	½ cup	100	1	0	0 [P]
Rosarita®, original, canned	½ cup	120	2	1	0
Rosarita®, no fat, canned	½ cup	90	0	0	0 [P]
Vegetarian					
Bearitos®, no salt, Organic	½ cup	140	2.5	0	0
Bearitos®, Spicy, low fat, Organic	½ cup	140	2.5	0	0
Tofu					
Firm, raw	½ cup	183	1	2	0
Regular, raw	½ cup	94	6	1	0
Shirataki, noodles	4 oz	20	1	0	0
Silken, Mor-nu® light firm,	1 slice	31	1	0	0
Silken, Mor-nu®, firm	1 slice	52	2	0	0
Silken, Mor-nu®, soft	1 slice	46	2	0	0

Dry Beans, Peas and Tofu

Chol (mg)	Sod (mg)	Carb (g)	Fiber (g)	Sugar (g)	Prot (g)
0	353	18	↑6	0	6
0	1	22	↑8	0	8
5	440	25	↑7	8 HF	6
0	420	23	↑6	7	6
0	409	8	4	1	2
0	13	10	4	na	11
0	19	14	↑5	na	17
0	↑600	19	↑5	3	5
0	270	21	↑7	0	7
0	↑570	17	↑6	1	6
0	310	18	↑6	0	7
0	↑590	17	↑5	1	7
0	5	23	↑9	2	7
0	↑540	24	↑9	2	8
0	18	5	3	na	20
0	9	2	0	na	10
0	15	3	2	0	1
0	71	1	0	na	5
0	30	2	0	1	6
0	4	2	0	1	4

The Meat and Bean Group | 91

Nuts, Nut Butters and Seeds

Nuts, Nut Butters and Seeds are considered part of the USDA Food Pyramid Meat and Bean Group.

USDA Recommendations:

Go lean on protein.

KEEP IT SIMPLE

Eat a total of 5.5 ounces per day— from the entire Meat and Bean Group. *USDA recommended Daily Serving is based on a 2,000 calorie diet.*

Nuts and Seeds are good source of **fiber,** vitamin E, calcium, potassium, phosphorous and more. They **do not contain cholesterol** and are naturally **low in sodium** and sugar.

Nuts and Seeds are ↑ **in fat** (mostly unsaturated "healthy" fat). Smaller servings are recommended since fat is a nutrient that needs to be limited.

Many nut and seed "butters," such as peanut butter or sesame butter, have **Trans Fats.** Compare the different kinds of Peanut Butters in this guide and on grocery store shelves. Look for brands that don't contain Partially Hydrogenated Oils.

Nuts and Seeds provide various health benefits. Walnuts and Flaxseed contain heart healthy Omega-3 essential fatty acids, and almonds are known for lowering bad cholesterol levels. Recognizing the benefits, the FDA approved the following health claim for whole or chopped nuts:

> "Scientific evidence suggests but does not prove that eating 1.5 ounces per day of most nuts as part of a diet low in saturated fat and cholesterol may reduce the risk of heart disease."

But, before going nuts, understand that nuts are high in calories. If you're watching your weight, nuts are not your best bet. If you have high blood pressure, limit salty nuts or nuts fried in oil.

EAT SMART. Enjoy the benefits by choosing raw nuts and seeds over salted, oil-roasted, honey, chocolate or yogurt coated varieties. Check the NUTRITION FACTS label for Trans Fats content and the INGREDIENTS list for "partially hydrogenated" oil to avoid Trans Fats. Try Organic Butters. Organic foods/products do *not* contain Trans Fat. Remember to eat all fat sparingly.

Item	Serving	Cal	Total Fat (g)	Sat Fat (g)	Trans Fat (g)

NUTS, NUT BUTTERS and SEEDS

Acorns
Dried	1 oz	144	9	1	0
Raw	1 oz	110	7	1	0

Almonds
Blanched	1 oz	165	↑14	1	0
Paste	1 oz	130	8	1	0
Raw	1 oz	164	↑14	1	0
Dry-roasted, with salt	1 oz	169	↑15	1	0
Honey-roasted	1 oz	168	↑14	1	0
Oil-roasted, with salt	1 oz	172	↑16	1	0
Smoked, Blue Diamond®, Smokehouse®	1 oz	170	↑16	1	0
Smoked, Blue Diamond®, Jalapeno flavor	1 oz	170	↑15	1	0

Almond Butter
Raw, Mara Natha®, Organic, no salt	1 tbsp	98	8	1	0
with salt	1 tbsp	101	9	1	0
no salt	1 tbsp	101	9	1	0
Beechnuts, dried	1 oz	163	↑14	2	0
Brazil nuts, dried	1 oz	186	↑19	↑4	0

Cashews
Raw	1 oz	157	12	2	0
Dry-roasted, with salt	1 oz	163	↑13	3	0
Honey-roasted, Planters®	1 oz	150	12	2	0
Oil-roasted, with salt	1 oz	165	↑14	2	0

Cashew Butter
with salt	1 tbsp	94	8	2	na
no salt	1 tbsp	94	8	2	na

Chestnuts
Chinese, dried	1 oz	103	1	0	0
Chinese, raw	1 oz	64	0	0	0
European, raw, peeled	1 oz	56	0	0	0
European, raw, unpeeled	1 oz	60	1	0	0
Japanese, raw	1 oz	44	0	0	0
Japanese, roasted	1 oz	57	0	0	0

Chol (mg)	Sod (mg)	Carb (g)	Fiber (g)	Sugar (g)	Prot (g)
0	0	15	na	na	2
0	0	12	na	na	2
0	8	6	3	1	6
0	3	14	1	10	3
0	0	6	3	1	6
0	96	5	3	1	6
0	37	8	4	na	5
0	96	5	3	1	6
0	150	5	3	1	6
0	180	5	3	1	6
0	0	3	2	1	4
0	72	3	1	1	2
0	2	3	1	1	2
0	11	10	na	na	2
0	1	3	2	1	4
0	3	9	1	2	5
0	181	9	1	1	4
0	85	11	1	4	4
0	87	9	1	1	5
0	98	4	1	1	3
0	2	4	1	na	3
0	1	23	1	na	2
0	1	14	na	na	1
0	1	13	na	na	0
0	1	13	2	na	1
0	4	10	na	na	1
0	5	13	na	na	1

The Meat and Bean Group

Item	Serving	Cal	Total Fat (g)	Sat Fat (g)	Trans Fat (g)
Coconut					
Cream, canned	1 tbsp	36	3	3	0
Meat, dried, flakes, sweetened	1 oz	129	8	↑7	0
Meat, Let's Do Organic®, dried, large flakes	3 tbsp	110	10	↑9	0
Meat, raw – 2"piece	1	159	↑15	↑13	0
Milk, canned	1 tbsp	30	3	3	0
Flaxseed, dried, whole	1 tbsp	55	4	0	0
Ginkgo Nuts					
Canned	1 oz	31	0	0	0
Dried	1 oz	99	1	0	0
Raw	1 oz	52	0	0	0
Hazelnuts (filbert)					
Raw	1 oz	178	↑17	1	0
Dry-roasted, with salt	1 oz	183	↑18	1	0
Hickory Nuts, dried	1 oz	186	↑18	2	0
Lotus Seeds					
Dried	1 oz	94	1	0	0
Raw	1 oz	25	0	0	0
Macadamia Nuts					
Butter, Mara Natha®	2 tbsp	230	↑24	↑4	0
Dry-roasted, with salt	1 oz	203	↑23	3	
Raw	1 oz	204	↑21	3	0
Mixed Nuts					
Dry-roasted, with salt	1 oz	168	↑15	2	0
NUT-rition, Planters®, Heart Healthy Mix	1 oz	170	↑16	1.5	0
Oil-roasted, with salt	1 oz	175	↑16	2	
Pecans					
Raw	1 oz	196	↑20	2	0
Dry-roasted, with salt	1 oz	201	↑21	2	
Oil-roasted, with salt	1 oz	203	↑21	2	
Peanuts					
All types, raw	1 oz	161	↑14	2	0
Dry-roasted, with salt	1 oz	166	↑14	2	
Honey-roasted, Planters®	1 oz	160	↑13	2	0

Chol (mg)	Sod (mg)	Carb (g)	Fiber (g)	Sugar (g)	Prot (g)
0	10	2	0	1	1
0	81	15	3	10	1
0	5	4	2	1	1
0	9	7	4	3	2
0	2	0	na	na	0
0	3	3	3	0	2
0	87	6	3	na	1
0	4	21	na	na	3
0	2	11	na	na	1
0	0	5	3	1	4
0	0	5	3	1	4
0	0	5	2	na	na
0	1	18	na	na	4
0	0	5	na	na	1
0	0	4	3	1	2
0	75	4	2	1	2
0	1	4	2	1	2
0	190	7	3	1	5
0	40	5	3	1	6
0	119	6	3	1	5
0	0	4	3	1	3
0	109	4	3	1	3
0	111	4	3	1	3
0	5	5	2	1	7
0	230	6	2	1	7
0	115	8	2	5	6

The Meat and Bean Group

Item	Serving	Cal	Total Fat (g)	Sat Fat (g)	Trans Fat (g)
Peanut Butter					
Crunchy, Jif®, extra crunchy	2 tbsp	190	↑16	3	0 [H,P]
Crunchy, Mara Natha®, Organic, no salt added	2 tbsp	190	↑16	2	0
Crunchy Skippy®, Super Chunk	2 tbsp	190	↑16	3	0 [P]
Creamy, Jif®, original	2 tbsp	190	↑16	3	0 [H,P]
Creamy, Jif®, reduced fat	2 tbsp	190	12	2.5	0 [H]
Creamy, Mara Natha®, no salt added	2 tbsp	190	↑16	2	0
Creamy, Skippy®, original	2 tbsp	190	↑16	3	0 [P]
Creamy, Skippy®, reduced fat	2 tbsp	190	12	2.5	0 [P]
Pine Nuts					
Dried	1 oz	191	↑19	1	0
Pinyon, dried	1 oz	178	↑17	3	0
Pistachios					
Raw	1 oz	158	↑13	2	0
Dry-roasted, with salt	1 oz	161	↑13	2	0
Pumpkin Seeds					
Dried, seed kernels	1 oz	153	↑13	2	0
Roasted, seed kernels	1 oz	148	12	2	0
Sesame					
Butter, Tahini, from raw kernels	1 tbsp	86	7	1	na
Butter, Tahini, from roasted kernels	1 tbsp	89	8	1	na
Paste	1 tbsp	94	8	1	na
Seeds, whole, raw	1 tbsp	52	4	1	0
Seeds, whole, roasted	1 oz	160	↑14	2	0
Sunflower					
Butter, with salt	1 tbsp	93	8	1	na
Seeds, dried, hulled, kernels	¼ cup	205	↑18	2	0
Seeds, dry-roasted, with salt	¼ cup	186	↑16	2	0
Seeds, oil-roasted, with salt	¼ cup	200	↑17	2	0
Walnuts					
Black, dried	1 oz	175	↑17	1	0
English	1 oz	185	↑18	2	0

Chol (mg)	Sod (mg)	Carb (g)	Fiber (g)	Sugar (g)	Prot (g)
0	130	7	2	3	8
0	0	7	3	1	8
0	120	7	2	3	7
0	150	7	2	3	8
0	250	15	1	4	8
0	0	7	3	1	8
0	150	7	2	3	7
0	190	15	2	5	7
0	1	4	1	1	4
0	20	5	3	na	3
0	0	8	3	2	6
0	115	8	3	2	6
0	5	5	1	0	7
0	163	4	1	1	9
0	11	4	1	na	3
0	17	3	1	0	3
0	2	4	1	na	3
0	1	2	1	0	2
0	3	7	4	na	5
0	83	4	na	na	3
0	1	7	4	1	8
0	131	8	3	1	6
0	138	8	4	1	6
0	1	3	2	1	7
0	1	4	2	1	4

The Meat and Bean Group

Beef, Pork and Lamb

Beef, Pork and **Lamb** is part of the USDA Food Pyramid Meat and Bean Group.

USDA Recommendations:

Go lean on protein.

KEEP IT SIMPLE

Eat a total of 5.5 ounces per day— from the entire Meat and Bean Group. *USDA recommended Daily Serving is based on a 2,000 calorie diet.*

Beef, Pork and Lamb can be ↑ **in fat,** ↑ **saturated fat and** ↑ **cholesterol.** Smaller servings are recommended.

Higher amounts of **sodium** are found in meat products that are cured, flavored or "enhanced." Enhanced products are injected with a solution (broth, sodium phosphate, etc.), marinated or basted.

Packaged Ground Meats, such as hamburger, may specify the percentage of lean meat vs. fat meat; however, may not provide total fat content.

Example:

80/20 = 80% lean meat / 20% fat

A six ounce serving of 80/20 is approximately 30 fat grams and 11 grams of saturated fat— almost 50% of the recommended Daily Value of fat. Compare different varieties of Ground Beef in this guide to make better choice.

There are three primary USDA grades of meat: Prime, Choice and Select.

USDA Prime— highest quality, highest in fat, lots of marbling (flecks of fat), most tender, juicy, used mostly by hotels and restaurants.

USDA Choice— most popular, less marbling (fat) than Prime, very tender, juicy, most widely sold at retail supermarkets.

USDA Select— leaner quality, lower in fat, fairly tender, increasing in popularity, found at most Meat counters.

Go to the "Beef" section in this chapter, locate "Loin," then "Tenderloin." Compare the fat content in prime tenderloin vs. select tenderloin. (Did you notice the difference?) Select tenderloin is 10 grams lower in fat than prime tenderloin.

Compare other cuts of meats in this guide to find lower fat options.

EAT SMART. The recommended serving of meat for a healthful meal is 3–4 ounces. A 3 ounce serving of meat is equal to one deck of cards. Many restaurants serve prime (high fat) meats 12 ounces or larger and can be shared. Remember the recommended Daily Value for the entire Meat and Bean Group is 5.5 ounces, based on a 2,000 calorie diet.

The Meat and Bean Group

Item	Serving	Cal	Total Fat (g)	Sat Fat (g)	Trans Fat (g)

BEEF

Brisket

Item	Serving	Cal	Total Fat (g)	Sat Fat (g)	Trans Fat (g)
Brisket, cooked	6 oz	687	↑58	↑23	0
Corned beef brisket, cooked	6 oz	427	↑32	↑11	0

Chuck

Item	Serving	Cal	Total Fat (g)	Sat Fat (g)	Trans Fat (g)
Eye steak, cooked	6 oz	272	9	3	0
Ground – 80/20, cooked	6 oz	462	↑30	↑11	2
Roast (blade), Choice, cooked	6 oz	617	↑47	↑18	0
Roast (blade), Prime, cooked	6 oz	709	↑58	↑24	0
Roast (blade), Select, cooked	6 oz	554	↑40	↑16	0
Flank, cooked	6 oz	321	↑13	↑5	0

Ground, Beef

Item	Serving	Cal	Total Fat (g)	Sat Fat (g)	Trans Fat (g)
70/30, crumbled, fresh, cooked	6 oz	459	↑30	↑12	1
75/25, crumbled, fresh, cooked	6 oz	471	↑31	↑12	2
80/20, crumbled, fresh, cooked	6 oz	462	↑30	↑11	2
85/15, crumbled, fresh, cooked	6 oz	435	↑26	↑10	2
90/10, crumbled, fresh, cooked	6 oz	391	↑20	↑8	1
95/05, crumbled, fresh, cooked	6 oz	328	↑13	↑6	0
Patty, Applegate Farms®, Organic, frozen	1	195	12	↑5	0
Patty, Laura's Lean®, frozen	1	160	9	↑4	0
Patty, Moran's® Big Patty, frozen	1	470	↑41	↑15	2.5
Jerky, Original, Golden Valley®, Organic	1 oz	70	1	0	0
Liver, calf	1 slice	130	4	1	0

Loin

Item	Serving	Cal	Total Fat (g)	Sat Fat (g)	Trans Fat (g)
New York Steak (shell steak), cooked	6 oz	449	↑29	↑11	0
Porterhouse, cooked	6 oz	559	↑44	↑17	0
T-bone, Choice, cooked	6 oz	547	↑42	↑17	0

Chol (mg)	Sod (mg)	Carb (g)	Fiber (g)	Sugar (g)	Prot (g)
↑156	110	0	0	0	38
↑167	↑1928	0	0	0	31
↑107	121	0	0	0	44
↑151	155	0	0	0	46
↑175	109	0	0	0	45
↑175	107	0	0	0	43
↑177	110	0	0	0	46
↑84	98	0	0	0	48
↑150	163	0	0	0	44
↑151	158	0	0	0	45
↑151	155	0	0	0	46
↑153	151	0	0	0	47
↑151	148	0	0	0	48
↑151	144	0	0	0	50
↑70	85	0	0	0	21
↑60	70	0	0	0	21
↑115	100	0	0	0	23
10	270	5	0	5	11
↑269	54	3	0	0	20
↑150	92	0	0	0	45
↑122	105	0	0	0	38
↑116	116	0	0	0	39

The Meat and Bean Group

Item	Serving	Cal	Total Fat (g)	Sat Fat (g)	Trans Fat (g)
Loin *continued*					
T-bone, Select, cooked	6 oz	478	↑33	↑13	0
Tenderloin (filet mignon), Choice	6 oz	464	↑30	↑12	0
Tenderloin (filet mignon), Prime	6 oz	524	↑38	↑15	0
Tenderloin (filet mignon), Select	6 oz	445	↑28	↑11	0
Top loin, cooked	6 oz	449	↑29	↑11	0
Rib					
Prime rib	6 oz	683	↑57	↑23	0
Rib eye steak	6 oz	403	↑24	↑9	0
Rib roast	6 oz	604	↑48	↑19	0
Round					
Eye round, cooked	6 oz	354	↑16	↑6	0
Ground round – 85/15, cooked	6 oz	435	↑26	↑10	2
London Broil, cooked	6 oz	371	↑20	↑8	0
Top round, cooked	6 oz	309	10	↑4	0
Skirt Steak	6 oz	374	↑20	↑8	0
Sirloin					
Ground – 90/10	6 oz	391	↑20	↑8	1
Top Sirloin, Choice	6 oz	437	↑27	↑11	0
Top Sirloin, Select	6 oz	391	↑22	↑9	0
Tri-Tip, Sirloin, Roast, cooked	6 oz	325	↑16	↑6	0
Veal					
Breast, boneless, cooked	6 oz	479	↑32	↑13	0
Ground, cooked	6 oz	292	↑13	↑5	0
Loin, cooked	6 oz	369	↑21	↑9	0
Sirloin, cooked	6 oz	343	↑18	↑8	0
Stew meat, cooked	6 oz	320	7	2	0
Beef, Dishes					
Pot Pie, Banquet®, frozen	1 pie	450	↑27	↑11	.5
BBQ Shredded Beef, Lloyds Barbeque Company®, Heat & Serve	¼ cup	90	1.5	.5	0 [P]
Tyson, Beef Tips, Heat & Serve	5 oz	200	12	↑4.5	0

Chol (mg)	Sod (mg)	Carb (g)	Fiber (g)	Sugar (g)	Prot (g)
↑102	112	0	0	0	42
↑158	88	0	0	0	45
↑146	100	0	0	0	43
↑148	97	0	0	0	45
↑150	92	0	0	0	45
↑144	107	0	0	0	38
↑181	91	0	0	0	44
↑144	109	0	0	0	39
↑105	63	0	0	0	48
↑153	151	0	0	0	47
↑128	60	0	0	0	45
↑110	68	0	0	0	55
↑102	128	0	0	0	44
↑151	148	0	0	0	48
↑141	92	0	0	0	46
↑114	97	0	0	0	46
↑121	92	0	0	0	43
↑190	109	0	0	0	44
↑175	141	0	0	0	41
↑175	158	0	0	0	42
↑173	141	0	0	0	43
↑246	158	0	0	0	59
30	↑730	36	2	7	14
15	390	11	1	9 HF	7
55	↑530	5	0	1	17

The Meat and Bean Group

Item	Serving	Cal	Total Fat (g)	Sat Fat (g)	Trans Fat (g)
Beef, Meals					
Banquet®					
Chicken Fried Steak, Hearty One, frozen	1 meal	750	↑42	↑14	2 [P]
Healthy Choice®					
Beef Tips Portobello, frozen	1 meal	300	8	2.5	0
Pot Roast, frozen	1 meal	310	7	3	0 [P]
Salisbury Steak, frozen	1 meal	360	9	↑3.5	0
Lean Cuisine®					
Beef Portobello, frozen	1 meal	220	6	2.5	0 [P]
Beef Pot Roast, frozen	1 meal	190	6	1.5	0
Peppercorn Beef, frozen	1 meal	220	7	2.5	0
South Beach®, Beef with Cheesy Broccoli	1 meal	240	7	↑3.5	0
Stouffer®					
Home Style Beef, Skillets, frozen	½ pkg	300	11	3	0
Meatloaf, Classic, frozen	1 meal	560	↑29	↑12	1.5 [P]
Pot Roast, Classic, frozen	1 meal	240	8	2.5	0

LAMB and GOAT

Item	Serving	Cal	Total Fat (g)	Sat Fat (g)	Trans Fat (g)
Lamb					
Ground, cooked	6 oz	481	↑33	↑14	0
Leg, Shank, bone-in, roasted	6 oz	369	↑19	↑8	0
Leg, Sirloin, bone-in, roasted	6 oz	483	↑33	↑14	0
Loin, roasted	6 oz	525	↑40	↑17	0
Goat					
Goat, Roasted	6 oz	243	5	2	0

PORK

Item	Serving	Cal	Total Fat (g)	Sat Fat (g)	Trans Fat (g)
Chops and Steaks					
Blade Chops, bone-in, broiled	6 oz	544	↑42	↑16	0
Blade Steaks, broiled	6 oz	440	↑28	↑10	0

Chol (mg)	Sod (mg)	Carb (g)	Fiber (g)	Sugar (g)	Prot (g)
↑59	↑1760	55	↑5	7	26
35	↑600	33	↑7	14 HF	20
45	↑500	45	↑5	21 HF	15
40	↑600	46	↑7	19 HF	20
30	↑660	25	2	6	16
25	↑690	22	3	4	13
25	↑690	25	3	8	14
↑90	↑910	16	4	7	26
40	↑1390	32	↑6	6	19
↑110	↑1180	40	↑8	10 HF	34
35	↑980	27	3	2	16

↑165	138	0	0	0	42
↑153	110	0	0	0	45
↑163	116	0	0	0	42
↑162	109	0	0	0	38
↑128	146	0	0	0	46

↑119	146	0	0	0	38
↑117	162	0	0	0	43

The Meat and Bean Group

Item	Serving	Cal	Total Fat (g)	Sat Fat (g)	Trans Fat (g)
Chops and Steaks *continued*					
Center Loin Chops, bone-in, broiled	6 oz	408	↑22	↑8	0
Sirloin Chops, bone-in, broiled	6 oz	440	↑27	↑10	0
Sirloin Chops, boneless, broiled	6 oz	354	↑15	↑5	0
Top Loin, boneless, broiled	6 oz	389	↑19	↑7	0
Top Loin, boneless, broiled, enhanced	6 oz	314	↑13	↑5	0
Ham					
Country Style, raw	6 oz	332	↑14	↑5	0
Extra-lean, cured, boneless, roasted	6 oz	246	9	3	0
Extra-lean, cured, boneless, roasted, canned	6 oz	231	8	3	0
Low-sodium, cured, bone-in, cured, cooked	6 oz	302	↑14	↑5	0
Rump, cured, bone-in, roasted	6 oz	270	↑14	↑5	0
Regular, cured, boneless, roasted, canned	6 oz	384	↑26	↑9	0
Shank, bone-in, roasted	6 oz	336	↑22	↑7	0
Steak, boneless, unheated	6 oz	208	7	2	0
Misc. Cuts					
Bacon, cured, cooked	2 slices	87	7	2	0
Bacon, Applegate Farms®, Sunday, Organic	2 slices	60	5	2	0
Bacon, Hormel®, Center Cut	2 slices	70	5	2	0
Bacon, Canadian, cured, cooked	2 slices	87	4	1	0
Bacon, Canadian, Applegate Farms®, uncured	2 slices	90	4	1.5	0
Ground Pork, cooked	6 oz	505	↑35	↑13	0
Loin filets, Hormel®, Lemon-Garlic flavor,	6 oz	198	7	2	0
Pancetta, Applegate Farms®	2 slices	90	7	2	0

Chol (mg)	Sod (mg)	Carb (g)	Fiber (g)	Sugar (g)	Prot (g)
↑139	99	0	0	0	49
↑146	116	0	0	0	45
↑155	95	0	0	0	52
↑138	107	0	0	0	51
↑124	338	0	0	0	47
↑119	↑4584	1	0	0	47
↑90	↑2045	3	0	0	36
51	↑1930	1	0	0	36
↑123	↑1431	1	0	1	43
↑106	↑1850	0	0	1	34
↑105	↑1600	1	0	0	35
11	↑1660	0	0	1	31
↑77	↑2159	0	0	0	33
18	370	0	0	0	6
10	290	0	0	0	4
15	300	0	0	0	5
27	↑727	1	0	0	11
35	↑500	1	0	1	12
↑160	124	0	0	0	44
↑71	↑991	3	0	0	30
25	460	0	0	0	6

The Meat and Bean Group

Item	Serving	Cal	Total Fat (g)	Sat Fat (g)	Trans Fat (g)
Misc. Cuts *continued*					
Prosciutto, Applegate Farms®, uncured	2 slices	70	4	1.5	0
Pork Tenderloin	6 oz	294	10	↑4	0
Pork Tenderloin, Hormel®, Peppercorn flavor, boneless, fresh	6 oz	185	6	2	0
Ribs					
Back ribs, roasted	6 oz	629	↑50	↑19	0
BBQ Baby back ribs, Lloyds Barbeque Company	2 ribs	290	↑17	↑7	0 [P]
Country Style, roasted	6 oz	558	↑43	↑16	0
Spareribs, cooked	6 oz	675	↑51	↑19	0
Pork Roasts					
Blade, Loin, bone-in	6 oz	547	↑42	↑16	0
Center Loin, bone-in, roasted	6 oz	398	↑23	↑9	0
Loin, Hormel®, boneless, fresh	6 oz	244	12	↑5	0
Top loin, boneless	6 oz	334	↑19	↑7	0
Picnic roast	6 oz	539	↑41	↑15	0
Sirloin, bone-in	6 oz	444	↑27	↑10	0
Sausage					
Ground					
Pork, Jimmy Dean®, Regular, ground roll	2 oz	220	↑21	↑7	0
Pork, Jimmy Dean®, ground roll, 50% less fat	2.5 oz	170	↑13	↑4.5	0
Pork, Jimmy Dean®, Maple, ground roll	2 oz	210	↑21	↑7	0
Pork, Owens®, Regular, ground roll	2 oz	180	↑15	↑6	0
Links					
Italian, Pork, link, cooked	1 link	286	↑23	↑8	0
Pork, Farmer John®, link	2 links	140	12	↑4	0
Pork, Oscar Mayer®, link	2 links	165	↑15	↑5	0
Smoked, Pork, link	1 link	265	↑22	↑8	0

Chol (mg)	Sod (mg)	Carb (g)	Fiber (g)	Sugar (g)	Prot (g)
25	↑570	0	0	0	2
↑134	94	0	0	0	47
↑79	↑998	3	0	0	29
↑201	172	0	0	0	41
↑70	↑850	20	1	19 HF	14
↑156	88	0	0	0	40
↑206	158	0	0	0	49
↑158	51	0	0	0	40
↑136	107	0	0	0	45
↑82	↑601	1	0	0	32
↑133	75	0	0	0	49
↑160	119	0	0	0	40
↑148	102	0	0	0	49
40	280	0	0	0	7
50	450	1	0	0	12
40	190	0	0	0	7
30	350	0	0	0	11
47	↑1002	4	0	1	16
30	400	1	0	0	6
37	401	0	0	0	8
46	↑1020	1	0	0	15

The Meat and Bean Group

Item	Serving	Cal	Total Fat (g)	Sat Fat (g)	Trans Fat (g)
Pork, Dishes					
BBQ Shredded Pork, Lloyd's Barbeque Company®, Heat & Serve	5 oz	90	1.5	.5	0 ᴾ
Pork Chops with Gravy, Hormel®, Heat & Serve	5 oz	160	6	2.5	0
Pork Roast in Gravy, Tyson®, Heat & Eat	5 oz	190	10	⬆4	0
Pork, Meals					
South Beach®, Savory Pork with Pecans & Green Beans	1 meal	240	10	2.5	0
Hungry Man®, Boneless Pork, 1 lb meal	1 meal	930	⬆49	15	0 ᴾ

Chol (mg)	Sod (mg)	Carb (g)	Fiber (g)	Sugar (g)	Prot (g)
15	400	11	0	9 HF	7
55	↑750	3	0	2	22
55	↑590	5	0	1	19
↑70	↑700	13	4	na	23
↑85	↑1940	↑106	4	65 HF	24

Lunch Meats, Sausage and Franks

Lunch Meats, Sausage and Franks are part of the USDA Food Pyramid Meat and Bean group.

USDA Recommendations:

Go lean on protein.

KEEP IT SIMPLE

Eat a total of 5.5 ounces per day— from the entire Meat and Bean Group. *USDA recommended Daily Serving is based on a 2,000 calorie diet.*

Lunch Meat, Sausage and Franks can be ↑ **in fat,** ↑ **saturated fat and** ↑ **in sodium.** Some contain 20% to 50% of your Daily Value of **sodium.**

Animal derived products, such as these, contain **cholesterol.**

EAT SMART. Choose lean or low fat lunch meats, sausage and franks or limit your serving size. Compare sodium on similar products.

Item	Serving	Cal	Total Fat (g)	Sat Fat (g)	Trans Fat (g)
LUNCH MEATS					
Bologna					
Bar-S®, original	1	100	8	2.5	na
Farmer John®, original	2 oz	160	↑14	↑4.5	.5
Oscar Mayer®, original	1	90	8	3	na
Beef, National Hebrew®, Kosher	1	80	8	↑3.5	0
Beef, Oscar Mayer®	1	90	8	↑3.5	0
Cheese, Oscar Mayer®	1	90	8	↑3.5	0
Light, Oscar Mayer®, 98% fat free	1	25	.5	0	0
Turkey, Bar-S®	1	60	4.5	1.5	0
Chicken, Oscar Mayer®, oven roasted, thin sliced	5	50	1	0	0
Ham					
Di Lusso®, Deluxe, Deli	2 oz	50	1	.5	0
Farmer John®, Premium sliced	2	50	1.5	1	0
Black Forest, Farmer John®, Premium 4x6	1	35	1	.5	0
Black Forest, Hormel®, Natural Choice	2 oz	60	2	na	0
Brown Sugar, Farmer John®, Brown Sugar & Honey 4x6	1	45	1	.5	0
Honey, Hormel®, Natural Choice	4 slices	70	2	1	0
Honey, Oscar Mayer®	6 slices	60	1.5	.5	0
Virginia, Hormel®, Natural Choice	2 oz	60	2	na	0
Head Cheese					
Farmer John®, sliced	1	100	7	↑4	0
Liverwurst					
Liverwurst, spread	2 oz	168	↑14	↑5	na
Olive Loaf					
Dietz & Watson®	2 oz	120	8	2.5	na
Pastrami					
Beef, cured	2 oz	82	2	1.5	na
Turkey	2 oz	70	2	1	na

Chol (mg)	Sod (mg)	Carb (g)	Fiber (g)	Sugar (g)	Prot (g)
35	350	2	0	1	3
25	↑520	2	0	1	6
30	300	1	0	1	3
15	240	0	0	0	3
20	310	1	1	1	3
20	320	1	0	0	3
10	240	3	0	1	3
25	370	3	0	1	3
25	↑520	1	0	1	9
25	↑670	2	0	2	9
20	↑700	1	0	0	10
15	↑470	1	0	0	7
35	↑530	0	0	0	11
15	410	2	0	2	7
25	↑550	3	0	3	9
35	↑800	2	0	2	11
35	↑530	0	0	0	11
30	400	0	0	0	8
↑65	385	3	1	1	7
20	↑580	7	0	7	6
38	↑496	0	0	0	12
39	↑559	2	0	2	9

The Meat and Bean Group | 117

Item	Serving	Cal	Total Fat (g)	Sat Fat (g)	Trans Fat (g)
Pepperoni					
Sandwich Style, Boar's Head®, Deli	1 oz	130	11	⬆4.5	na
Turkey Pepperoni, Hormel®	17 slices	80	4	1.5	0
Prosciutto					
Boar's Head®, Deli	1 oz	60	3	1	na
Roast Beef					
Hormel®, Naturals, Deli	4 slices	70	2.5	1	0
Oscar Mayer®, Deli, Slow Roasted, shaved	6 slices	60	2.5	1	0
Salami, Cotto					
Bar-S®	1	90	8	2.5	0
Farmer John®	1	140	1	⬆4	0
Spam	2 oz	180	⬆16	⬆6	0
Spam, light	2 oz	110	8	2	0
Turkey					
Bar-S®, Turkey Breast, extra lean	1	35	.5	0	0
Farmer John®, Turkey Breast, Roasted	1 slice	25	0	0	0
Oscar Mayer®, Turkey Breast, Smoked, shaved	6 slices	60	1	0	0

SAUSAGE and FRANKS

Item	Serving	Cal	Total Fat (g)	Sat Fat (g)	Trans Fat (g)
Bratwurst					
Beef & Pork, smoked	2 oz	196	⬆16	⬆4	na
Chicken, cooked	3 oz	148	9	⬆9	na
Pork, cooked	3 oz	283	⬆25	⬆9	na
Turkey, Jennie-O®	1	170	9	⬆10	2
Chorizo					
Pork & Beef, 4 inch link	1	273	⬆23	⬆9	na
Frankfurters					
Bar-S®, original	1	120	11	⬆3.5	0
Bar-S®, Jumbo	1	170	⬆14	⬆4.5	0
Beef, Bar-S®, original	1	130	12	⬆5	0
Beef, Bar-S®, Jumbo	1	180	⬆16	⬆7	0
Beef, Farmer John®, Premium Jumbo	1	180	⬆16	⬆8	1

Lunch Meats, Sausage and Franks

Chol (mg)	Sod (mg)	Carb (g)	Fiber (g)	Sugar (g)	Prot (g)
25	↑480	1	0	1	6
40	↑600	0	0	0	9
15	↑750	0	0	0	8
25	↑500	0	0	0	11
30	↑520	0	0	0	10
40	360	2	0	1	3
45	↑470	3	0	1	7
40	↑790	1	0	0	7
40	↑580	1	0	0	9
15	350	2	0	1	5
10	270	1	0	1	5
20	↑630	2	0	0	9

51	↑560	1	0	0	8
↑60	60	0	0	0	16
↑63	↑719	2	0	0	12
↑70	↑670	2	0	2	17
53	↑741	1	0	0	14
40	↑480	3	0	1	4
55	↑640	4	0	2	5
30	450	1	0	0	5
35	↑600	1	0	0	7
35	↑650	2	0	2	6

The Meat and Bean Group | 119

Item	Serving	Cal	Total Fat (g)	Sat Fat (g)	Trans Fat (g)
Frankfurters *continued*					
Beef, Farmer John®, Premium Quarter Pounder	1	350	↑31	↑11	1.5
Beef, Hebrew National®, Kosher	1	150	↑14	↑6	0
Beef, Hebrew National®, 97% fat free, Kosher	1	45	1.5	1	0
Beef, Oscar Mayer®, Jumbo	1	180	↑17	↑7	1
Chicken, Bar-S®	1	110	9	3	0
Turkey, Bar-S®, Jumbo	1	120	9	2.5	0
Hot Dogs/Weiners					
Oscar Mayer®, original	1	130	12	↑4	0
Oscar Mayer®, Bun Length	1	170	↑16	↑5	0
Oscar Mayer®, 98% Fat Free	1	40	0	0	0
Oscar Mayer®, Turkey	1	100	8	2.5	0
Corn Dogs					
Bar-S®	1	240	↑15	↑4	0
Farmer John®, Premium	1	220	12	↑4	0
Kielbasa					
Turkey & Beef, Polish, smoked	2 oz	127	10	3	na

Chol (mg)	Sod (mg)	Carb (g)	Fiber (g)	Sugar (g)	Prot (g)
↑75	↑1150	5	0	1	13
30	370	1	0	0	6
15	400	3	0	0	6
35	↑580	2	0	1	6
50	440	4	0	2	4
50	↑680	4	0	2	6
35	↑540	1	0	1	5
45	↑680	1	0	0	6
15	↑470	3	0	1	5
30	↑510	2	0	1	5
50	↑620	23	0 [E]	7	5
25	↑530	19	1 [E]	5	7
39	↑672	2	0	0	7

The Meat and Bean Group

Poultry

Poultry, including **Chicken, Duck, Goose** and **Turkey,** is part of the USDA Food Pyramid Meat and Bean Group.

USDA Recommendations:

Go lean on protein.

KEEP IT SIMPLE

Eat a total of 5.5 ounces per day— from the entire Meat and Bean Group. *USDA recommended Daily Serving is based on a 2,000 calorie diet.*

Poultry is a good source of protein and tends to be **lower in fat** and **cholesterol** than other Meats.

Poultry can be ↑ **in fat,** ↑ **saturated fat** and ↑ **in cholesterol,** depending on what you choose.

White poultry meat is known for being lower in fat than dark poultry meat. In fact, white meat has half the amount of fat and saturated fat than dark meat.

Eating the skin? Poultry with skin is just as **high in fat** and **saturated fat** as many beef and pork products.

Check out the examples of poultry with and without skin:

> **White meat** (skinless, chicken) =
> 8 grams of fat / 2 grams of saturated fat
>
> **Dark meat** (skinless, chicken) =
> 16 grams of fat / 4 grams of saturated fat
>
> **White meat** (with skin, chicken) =
> 13 grams of fat / 4 grams of saturated fat
>
> **Dark meat** (with skin, chicken) =
> 27 grams of fat / 7 grams of saturated fat

Breaded or fried poultry is generally ↑ **in fat** and ↑ **sodium** and may contain refined carbohydrates due to the use of white or wheat flour. Removing the skin will help reduce total fat.

Higher amounts of sodium are found in enhanced, flavored, marinated or basted products as well frozen meals and canned poultry.

EAT SMART. Choose white skinless meat more often. Grill, bake or broil poultry. Limit breaded or fried poultry. Season Poultry with herbs or low fat, low sodium marinades. Consider topping Poultry with pico—fresh chopped tomatoes, cilantro, onions and jalapenos instead of cream based or high fat sauces.

Item	Serving	Cal	Total Fat (g)	Sat Fat (g)	Trans Fat (g)

CHICKEN

Breasts
Item	Serving	Cal	Total Fat (g)	Sat Fat (g)	Trans Fat (g)
Fried, skinless	6 oz	314	8	2	0
Lemon Herb, Foster Farms®, skinless	1 filet	220	3	0	0
Roasted, skinless	6 oz	277	6	2	0
with skin, fried	6 oz	437	↑22	6	0
with skin, roasted	6 oz	328	↑13	↑4	0

Canned
Item	Serving	Cal	Total Fat (g)	Sat Fat (g)	Trans Fat (g)
White meat, Swanson®	6 oz	150	3	1.5	0
White meat, Valley Fresh®	6 oz	210	3	0	0
White & Dark meat, Valley Fresh®	6 oz	240	6	1.5	0

Cornish Game Hen
Item	Serving	Cal	Total Fat (g)	Sat Fat (g)	Trans Fat (g)
Skinless, roasted	1	295	9	2	0
with skin, roasted	1	668	↑47	↑13	0

Dark Meat
Item	Serving	Cal	Total Fat (g)	Sat Fat (g)	Trans Fat (g)
Fried, skinless	6 oz	402	↑20	↑5	0
Roasted, skinless	6 oz	344	↑16	↑4	0
with skin, fried	6 oz	591	↑31	↑8	0
with skin, roasted	6 oz	425	↑27	↑7	0

Drum Stick
Item	Serving	Cal	Total Fat (g)	Sat Fat (g)	Trans Fat (g)
Fried, skinless	1	82	3	1	0
Roasted, skinless	1	76	2	1	0
with skin, fried	1	193	11	3	0
with skin, roasted	1	112	6	2	0
Giblets, cooked	4 oz	120	4	1	0

Leg
Item	Serving	Cal	Total Fat (g)	Sat Fat (g)	Trans Fat (g)
Fried, skinless	1	196	9	2	0
Roasted, skinless	1	181	8	2	0
with skin, fried	1	431	↑26	↑7	0
with skin, roasted	1	264	↑15	↑4	0

Light Meat
Item	Serving	Cal	Total Fat (g)	Sat Fat (g)	Trans Fat (g)
Fried, skinless	6 oz	322	9	3	0
Roasted, skinless	6 oz	291	8	2	0
with skin, fried	6 oz	465	↑26	↑7	0

Chol (mg)	Sod (mg)	Carb (g)	Fiber (g)	Sugar (g)	Prot (g)
↑153	136	1	0	0	57
↑130	↑720	8	0	8	40
↑143	127	0	0	0	52
↑143	↑462	15	0	0	42
↑140	118	0	0	0	50
↑60	↑810	3	0	3	30
↑75	↑540	0	0	0	45
↑150	180	0	0	0	45
↑223	139	0	0	0	51
↑337	164	0	0	0	57
↑161	163	4	0	0	47
↑156	156	0	0	0	45
↑150	↑496	16	0	0	37
↑153	146	0	0	0	48
4	39	0	0	0	12
41	42	0	0	0	12
↑62	194	6	0	0	16
47	47	0	0	0	14
↑259	44	1	0	0	19
↑93	90	1	0	0	27
↑89	86	0	0	0	26
↑142	441	14	0	0	34
↑105	99	0	0	0	30
↑151	136	1	0	0	55
↑143	129	0	0	0	52
↑141	↑482	16	0	0	40

The Meat and Bean Group

Item	Serving	Cal	Total Fat (g)	Sat Fat (g)	Trans Fat (g)
Light Meat *continued*					
with skin, roasted	6 oz	373	↑18	↑5	0
Thigh					
Fried, skinless	1	113	5	1	0
Roasted, skinless	1	109	6	↑5	0
with skin, fried	1	238	↑14	↑4	0
with skin, roasted	1	153	10	3	0
Wing					
with skin, fried	1	159	11	3	0
with skin, roasted	1	99	7	2	0
Chicken, Dishes					
Pot Pies					
Applegate Farms®, Organic, frozen	1 pie	470	↑24	↑6	0
Marie Callender's®, Chicken Pot Pie, frozen	1 cup	520	↑520	↑9	1.5
Nuggets					
Breaded, Tyson's®, frozen bag	5	280	↑18	↑4	0
Honey BBQ shaped Wyngs, Tyson's®, Frozen bag	3	200	9	1.5	0
Misc. Chicken Dishes					
Chicken Parmigiana, Stouffer®, Family Size, frozen	1 piece	460	↑18	↑4	0
Chicken, Meals					
Birds Eye®					
Cheesy Chicken, Family Skillets, Frozen bag, cooked	1 cup	250	6	3	0 [P]
Garlic Chicken, Family Skillets, Frozen bag, cooked	1 cup	240	8	2	1 [P]
Healthy Choice®					
Chicken Margherita, frozen	1 meal	340	8	1.5	0
Chicken Parmigiana, frozen	1 meal	370	9	2	0
Chicken Teriyaki, frozen	1 meal	280	4	1	0
Mandarin Chicken, frozen	1 meal	240	2.5	.5	0 [P]

Chicken

Chol (mg)	Sod (mg)	Carb (g)	Fiber (g)	Sugar (g)	Prot (g)
↑141	126	0	0	0	48
53	49	1	0	0	15
49	46	0	0	0	13
↑80	248	8	0	0	19
↑58	52	0	0	0	16
39	157	5	0	0	10
29	28	0	0	0	9
30	↑760	50	2	10	14
25	↑800	44	3	5	14
40	↑480	16	0	0	14
20	↑740	19	0	3	13
35	↑1060	56	4	9	18
5	↑830	35	3	6	14
20	↑540	29	3	6	11
30	↑550	43	4	8	23
15	↑500	56	↑6	19 [HF]	16
25	↑550	44	↑8	25	15
15	↑510	39	↑5	9	13

The Meat and Bean Group

Item	Serving	Cal	Total Fat (g)	Sat Fat (g)	Trans Fat (g)
Chicken, Meals *continued*					
Hungry Man®					
Boneless Fried Chicken, 1 lb meal, frozen	1 meal	710	↑29	↑7	0
Kashi®					
Chicken Florentine, frozen	1 meal	290	9	↑4.5	0
Sweet and Sour Chicken, frozen	1 meal	320	3.5	.5	0
Lemon Rosemary Chicken, frozen	1 meal	330	9	1.5	0
Lean Cuisine®					
Chicken a L'orange, frozen	1 meal	260	3	.5	0
Grilled Chicken with Teriyaki Glaze, frozen	1 meal	270	3	1	0
Baked Chicken, frozen	1 meal	240	4.5	1	0 [P]
South Beach®, Garlic Herb Chicken with Green Beans	1 meal	270	11	2	0
Stouffer®, Teriyaki Chicken, Skillet, frozen bag	½ pkg	310	4.5	1	0 [P]

DUCK and GOOSE

Item	Serving	Cal	Total Fat (g)	Sat Fat (g)	Trans Fat (g)
Duck					
Skinless, roasted	6 oz	338	↑19	↑7	0
with skin, roasted	6 oz	566	↑48	↑16	0
Goose					
Skinless, roasted	6 oz	400	↑21	↑8	0
with skin, roasted	6 oz	512	↑37	↑12	0

TURKEY

Item	Serving	Cal	Total Fat (g)	Sat Fat (g)	Trans Fat (g)
Bacon					
Applegate Farms®, Organic	2 slices	70	2	0	0
Jennie O®, regular	2 slices	70	5	1	0
Breasts					
Roasted, skinless	6 oz	227	1	0	0
with skin, roasted	6 oz	257	5	1	0

Chol (mg)	Sod (mg)	Carb (g)	Fiber (g)	Sugar (g)	Prot (g)
↑165	↑2160	↑86	↑6	30	34
45	↑550	31	↑5 W	1	22
35	380	55	↑6 W	25	18
15	↑640	45	↑5 W	1	17
30	↑580	39	2	12 HF	18
40	↑660	42	0	11 HF	19
25	↑650	34	3	5 HF	19
↑65	↑660	13	4	3	28
50	↑1130	44	↑6	10	23

↑150	109	0	0	0	39
↑141	99	0	0	0	32
↑161	128	0	0	0	49
↑153	118	0	0	0	42

30	420	0	0	0	12
20	250	2	0	0	4
↑139	87	0	0	0	50
↑151	89	0	0	0	49

The Meat and Bean Group

Item	Serving	Cal	Total Fat (g)	Sat Fat (g)	Trans Fat (g)
Canned					
White meat, Valley Fresh®,	6 oz	240	4.5	1.5	0
Dark Meat					
Roasted, skinless	6 oz	314	12	↑4	0
with skin, roasted	6 oz	371	↑19	↑6	0
Gizzard, cooked	1	103	3	1	0
Ground					
Applegate Farms®, Organic, frozen patty	1 patty	170	8	2	0
Jennie O®, frozen burger	1 patty	250	↑17	↑4	0
Leg					
Roasted, skinless	1	356	8	3	0
with skin, roasted	1	416	↑13	↑4	0
Light Meat					
Roasted, skinless	6 oz	235	2	1	0
with skin, roasted	6 oz	276	8	2	0
Liver, cooked	1	227	↑17	↑6	0
Roast					
Boneless, light and dark meat, seasoned	6 oz	260	10	3	0
Turkey Breast Roast with Gravy, Jennie O®, Heat & Serve	4 oz	160	8	2	0
Wing					
Roasted, skinless	1	98	2	1	0
with skin, roasted	1	186	9	2	0
Turkey, Dishes					
Pot Pie, Banquet®, frozen	1 pie	380	↑21	↑9	0
Turkey, Meals					
Turkey, Banquet®, Healthy One, frozen	1 meal	430	↑16	↑4	0 [P]
Slow Roasted Turkey with Gravy, Healthy Choice®, frozen	1 meal	200	4	1	0 [P]

Chol (mg)	Sod (mg)	Carb (g)	Fiber (g)	Sugar (g)	Prot (g)
16	450	0	0	0	48
↑143	133	0	0	0	48
↑150	128	0	0	0	46
↑171	56	0	0	0	18
↑85	65	0	0	0	24
↑90	↑750	0	0	0	27
↑267	181	0	0	0	65
↑172	196	0	0	0	70
↑144	94	0	0	0	51
↑160	96	0	0	0	48
↑322	46	1	0	0	17
↑89	↑1142	5	0	0	36
↑60	↑770	3	0	2	19
↑61	47	0	0	0	19
↑104	66	0	0	0	25
35	↑840	36	2	3	10
50	↑2150	43	↑9	5	29
20	↑570	24	↑5	2	15

The Meat and Bean Group

Fish and Shellfish

Fish and Shellfish are part of the USDA Food Pyramid Meat and Bean Group.

USDA Recommendations:

Go lean on protein.

Vary your choices with more fish.

KEEP IT SIMPLE

Eat a total of 5.5 ounces per day— from the entire Meat and Bean Group. *USDA recommended Daily Serving is based on a 2,000 calorie diet.*

Fish and Shellfish are an important part of a healthy diet and an excellent source of protein.

Some fish contain heart healthy Omega-3 essential fatty acids. Wild cold water fish, such as salmon, herring and mackerel, are known to be ↑ **in "healthy"** Omega-3 **fat.** Choose these varieties more often. Smaller serving sizes are best.

The average serving size for fish is 3–6 ounces. To attain the health benefits, eat fish twice a week. Eating fish regularly may reduce the risk of heart disease.

Wild fish are **lower in fat** than farmed fish primarily due to diet and exercise. Compare wild and farmed fish in this chapter. You will notice a difference.

Breaded, fried or processed fish and shellfish are generally ↑ **in fat,** ↑ **sodium and** ↑**cholesterol,** and may contain small amounts of carbohydrates due to the use of flour.

Canned fish such as tuna is ↑ **in sodium.**

> **Mercury warning:** Women who might become pregnant, women who are pregnant, nursing mothers and young children should limit seafood consumption to reduce exposure to the harmful effect of mercury.

Shark, Swordfish, King Mackerel and Tilefish contain high levels of mercury and should be avoided.

Fish and Shellfish that have lower levels of mercury are shrimp, canned light tuna, salmon, pollock, and catfish and are better choices for women and children.

Dry heat cooking methods referenced in this chapter are grilling, broiling and baking.

EAT SMART. Grill, broil or bake fish. Limit breaded or fried fish/shellfish. Women and children should focus on fish and shellfish low in mercury. To reduce sodium—season Fish and Shellfish with lemon and herbs, such as dill, cilantro or salt free herb blends. Try low sodium or sodium free spices or marinades.

The Meat and Bean Group

Item	Serving	Cal	Total Fat (g)	Sat Fat (g)	Trans Fat (g)
FISH					
Anchovy, canned, in oil	1 oz	60	3	1	0
Bass					
Freshwater, cooked, dry heat	6 oz	248	8	2	0
Freshwater, raw	6 oz	194	6	1	0
Striped, cooked, dry heat	6 oz	211	5	1	0
Striped, raw	6 oz	165	4	1	0
Bluefish					
Cooked, dry heat	6 oz	270	9	2	0
Raw	6 oz	211	7	2	0
Burbot					
Cooked, dry heat	6 oz	196	2	0	0
Raw	6 oz	153	1	0	0
Butterfish					
Cooked, dry heat	6 oz	318	↑17	na	0
Raw	6 oz	248	↑14	↑6	0
Catfish, Channel					
Cooked, breaded & fried	6 oz	389	↑23	↑6	na
Farmed, cooked, dry heat	6 oz	258	↑14	3	0
Farmed, raw	6 oz	230	↑13	3	0
Wild, cooked, dry heat	6 oz	178	5	1	0
Wild, raw	6 oz	162	5	1	0
Cod					
Atlantic, cooked, dry heat	6 oz	178	1	0	0
Atlantic, raw	6 oz	139	1	0	0
Pacific, cooked, dry heat	6 oz	178	1	0	0
Pacific, raw	6 oz	139	1	0	0
Croaker, Atlantic					
Cooked, breaded & fried	6 oz	376	↑22	↑6	na
Raw	6 oz	177	5	2	0

Chol (mg)	Sod (mg)	Carb (g)	Fiber (g)	Sugar (g)	Prot (g)
24	↑1040	0	0	0	8
↑148	153	0	0	0	41
↑116	119	0	0	0	32
↑175	150	0	0	0	39
↑136	117	0	0	0	30
↑129	131	0	0	0	44
↑100	102	0	0	0	34
↑131	211	0	0	0	42
↑102	165	0	0	0	33
↑141	194	0	0	0	38
↑110	151	0	0	0	29
↑138	↑476	14	1	0	31
↑109	136	0	0	0	32
↑80	90	0	0	0	26
↑122	85	0	0	0	31
↑99	73	0	0	0	28
↑94	133	0	0	0	39
↑73	92	0	0	0	30
↑80	155	0	0	0	39
↑73	92	0	0	0	30
↑143	↑592	13	1	0	31
↑104	95	0	0	0	30

The Meat and Bean Group

Item	Serving	Cal	Total Fat (g)	Sat Fat (g)	Trans Fat (g)
Cusk					
Cooked, dry heat	6 oz	190	2	na	0
Raw	6 oz	148	1	0	0
Drum, Freshwater					
Cooked, dry heat	6 oz	260	11	2	0
Raw	6 oz	202	8	2	0
Eel					
Cooked, dry heat	6 oz	404	↑25	↑5	0
Raw	6 oz	313	↑20	↑4	0
Filets, Frozen					
Gorton's®					
Battered, Beer	2 fillets	230	↑14	2.5	0
Battered, Original	2 fillets	260	↑17	3	0
Breaded, Original	2 fillets	240	12	2.5	0
Breaded, Ranch	2 fillets	240	↑13	2.5	0
Grilled, Cajun Blackened	1 fillet	100	3	.5	0
Grilled, Char-Grilled	1 fillet	100	3	.5	0
Grilled, Lemon Butter	1 fillet	100	3	.5	0 [P]
Ian's®, Breaded, original	1 fillet	260	8	1	0
Van de Kamp's®					
Battered, Beer	1 fillet	120	6	1.5	0
Battered, Crispy Fish Tenders	4 pieces	210	10	↑3.5	0
Battered, Original	1 fillet	120	6	2	0
Breaded, Crisp & Healthy	2 fillets	150	1.5	1	0 [P]
Breaded, Original	2 fillets	230	↑13	↑4.5	0
Fish Sticks					
Breaded, Gorton's®	6 sticks	250	↑14	2.5	0
Breaded, Ian's®, gluten Free	5 sticks	190	6	1	0
Breaded, Ian's®, Original	5 sticks	190	6	1	0
Breaded, Van de Kamp's®, Crisp & Healthy	6 sticks	140	1	.5	0 [P]
Breaded, Van de Kamp's®	6 sticks	260	↑13	↑4.5	0

Chol (mg)	Sod (mg)	Carb (g)	Fiber (g)	Sugar (g)	Prot (g)
↑90	68	0	0	0	41
↑70	53	0	0	0	32
↑139	163	0	0	0	38
↑109	128	0	0	0	30
↑274	110	0	0	0	40
↑214	87	0	0	0	31
20	↑640	18	0 [E]	3	9
30	↑770	17	0 [E]	3	9
30	↑555	23	0 [E]	3	9
30	↑650	22	0 [E]	3	9
↑60	330	1	0	0	17
↑60	250	1	0	0	17
↑60	380	1	0	0	17
20	410	32	2	4	14
15	380	12	1 [E]	2	6
20	↑700	22	1 [E]	5	9
10	370	12	1 [E]	3	5
20	↑470	25	1 [E]	4	8
20	440	21	1 [E]	2	8
20	380	20	0 [E]	2	11
15	310	24	1	3	11
15	310	24	1	3	11
25	↑470	25	1 [E]	4	9
25	380	24	1 [E]	3	9

The Meat and Bean Group | 137

Item	Serving	Cal	Total Fat (g)	Sat Fat (g)	Trans Fat (g)
Grouper					
Cooked, dry heat	6 oz	201	2	1	0
Raw	6 oz	156	2	0	0
Haddock					
Cooked, dry heat	6 oz	190	2	0	0
Raw	6 oz	148	1	0	0
Halibut					
Cooked, dry heat	6 oz	238	5	1	0
Raw	6 oz	187	4	1	0
Herring					
Atlantic, cooked, dry heat	6 oz	345	↑20	↑4	0
Atlantic, raw	6 oz	296	↑15	3	0
Pacific, cooked, dry heat	6 oz	425	↑30	↑7	0
Pacific, raw	6 oz	332	↑24	↑6	0
Mackerel, King					
Cooked, dry heat	6 oz	228	4	1	0
Raw	6 oz	178	3	1	0
Perch					
Cooked, dry heat	6 oz	199	2	0	0
Raw	6 oz	155	2	0	0
Pollock					
Cooked, dry heat	6 oz	201	2	0	0
Raw	6 oz	156	2	0	0
Roughy, Orange					
Cooked, dry heat	6 oz	178	2	0	0
Raw	6 oz	129	1	0	0
Sable					
Cooked, dry heat	6 oz	425	↑33	↑7	0
Raw	6 oz	332	↑26	↑5	0
Salmon					
Atlantic, farmed, cooked	6 oz	350	↑21	↑4	0
Atlantic, farmed, raw	6 oz	311	↑18	↑4	0
Atlantic, wild, cooked	6 oz	309	↑14	2	0
Atlantic, wild, raw	6 oz	241	11	2	0

Chol (mg)	Sod (mg)	Carb (g)	Fiber (g)	Sugar (g)	Prot (g)
↑80	90	0	0	0	42
↑63	90	0	0	0	33
↑126	148	0	0	0	41
↑97	116	0	0	0	32
↑70	117	0	0	0	45
54	92	0	0	0	35
↑131	196	0	0	0	39
↑102	153	0	0	0	31
↑168	162	0	0	0	36
↑131	126	0	0	0	28
↑116	345	0	0	0	44
↑90	269	0	0	0	34
↑196	134	0	0	0	42
↑153	105	0	0	0	33
↑155	187	0	0	0	42
↑121	146	0	0	0	33
↑136	117	0	0	0	38
↑102	112	0	0	0	28
↑107	122	0	0	0	29
↑83	95	0	0	0	21
↑107	104	0	0	0	37
↑100	100	0	0	0	34
↑121	95	0	0	0	43
↑94	75	0	0	0	34

Item	Serving	Cal	Total Fat (g)	Sat Fat (g)	Trans Fat (g)
Salmon *continued*					
Chinook (king), cooked	6 oz	393	↑23	↑5	0
Chinook (king), raw	6 oz	304	↑18	↑5	0
Chinook (king), smoked	6 oz	199	7	2	0
Pink, canned	6 oz	231	8	1	0
Pink, cooked	6 oz	253	8	1	0
Pink, raw	6 oz	197	6	1	0
Sockeye (red), canned	6 oz	282	12	3	0
Sockeye (red), cooked	6 oz	367	↑19	3	0
Sockeye (red), raw	6 oz	286	↑15	3	0
Smoked Salmon, (Alaska native)	6 oz	556	↑19	↑4	0
Sardines					
Atlantic, canned in oil	4	100	6	1	0
Shad					
Cooked, dry heat	6 oz	428	↑30	na	0
Raw	6 oz	335	↑23	↑5	0
Snapper					
Cooked, dry heat	6 oz	218	3	1	0
Raw	6 oz	170	2	0	0
Swordfish					
Cooked, dry heat	6 oz	264	9	2	0
Raw	6 oz	206	7	2	0
Tilapia					
Cooked, dry heat	6 oz	218	5	2	0
Raw	6 oz	163	3	1	0
Breaded, Gorton's®, frozen	1 fillet	230	12	↑3.5	0
Breaded, Van de Camp's®, frozen	1 fillet	240	11	2.5	0
Trout, Rainbow					
Farmed, cooked, dry heat	6 oz	287	12	↑4	0
Farmed, raw	6 oz	235	9	3	0
Wild, cooked, dry heat	6 oz	255	10	3	0
Wild, raw	6 oz	202	6	1	0

Chol (mg)	Sod (mg)	Carb (g)	Fiber (g)	Sugar (g)	Prot (g)
↑144	102	0	0	0	43
↑85	80	0	0	0	34
39	↑1333	0	0	0	31
↑139	↑678	0	0	0	39
↑114	146	0	0	0	44
↑88	114	0	0	0	34
↑75	↑612	0	0	0	40
↑148	112	0	0	0	46
↑105	80	0	0	0	36
↑240	↑1700	0	0	0	97
↑68	242	0	0	0	12
↑163	110	0	0	0	37
↑128	87	0	0	0	29
↑80	97	0	0	0	45
↑63	109	0	0	0	35
↑85	196	0	0	0	43
↑66	153	0	0	0	33
↑97	95	0	0	0	44
↑85	88	0	0	0	34
25	420	20	1 [E]	1	11
35	280	17	1	1	16
↑116	71	0	0	0	41
↑100	60	0	0	0	35
↑117	95	0	0	0	39
↑100	53	0	0	0	35

The Meat and Bean Group

Item	Serving	Cal	Total Fat (g)	Sat Fat (g)	Trans Fat (g)
Tuna					
Blue fin	6 oz	313	11	3	0
Chunk Light, Bumble Bee®, canned in oil	6 oz	330	↑18	3	0
Chunk Light, Bumble Bee®, canned in water	6 oz	180	1.5	0	0
Chunk Light, Chicken of the Sea®, canned in oil	6 oz	330	↑18	3	0
Chunk Light, Chicken of the Sea®, canned in water	6 oz	180	1.5	0	0
Chunk Light, StarKist®, canned in water	6 oz	180	1.5	0	0
White (Albacore), Bumble Bee®, canned in oil	6 oz	270	9	3	0
White (Albacore), Chicken of the Sea®, canned in oil	6 oz	270	9	3	0
White (Albacore), Bumble Bee®, canned in water	6 oz	210	3	0	0
White (Albacore), Chicken of the Sea®, canned in water	6 oz	180	3	0	0
White (Albacore), StarKist®, canned in water	6 oz	210	3	0	0
Fish, Meals					
Healthy Choice®					
Herb Baked Fish	1 meal	360	8	2	0
Lemon Pepper Fish	1 meal	310	4.5	1	0
Salmon, Creamy Dill	1 meal	240	6	2.5	0
Lean Cuisine®					
Baked Lemon Pepper Fish	1 meal	230	6	2	0 [H, P]
Salmon with Lemon Dill Sauce	1 meal	240	6	2.5	0

Chol (mg)	Sod (mg)	Carb (g)	Fiber (g)	Sugar (g)	Prot (g)
↑83	85	0	0	0	51
↑90	↑750	0	0	0	39
↑90	↑750	0	0	0	39
↑90	↑750	0	0	0	39
↑90	↑750	0	0	0	39
↑90	↑750	0	0	0	39
↑75	↑750	0	0	0	42
↑75	↑750	0	0	0	42
↑75	↑750	0	0	0	45
↑75	↑750	0	0	0	39
↑75	↑750	0	0	0	45
40	↑590	55	5	13	16
20	440	53	5	14	13
15	↑600	26	5	1 HF	19
45	↑690	23	2	6	20
30	↑690	30	4	4	16

The Meat and Bean Group

Item	Serving	Cal	Total Fat (g)	Sat Fat (g)	Trans Fat (g)

SHELLFISH

Clam
Canned	6 oz	252	3	0	0
Cooked, battered & fried	6 oz	343	↑19	↑5	0
Cooked, steamed	6 oz	252	3	0	0

Crab
Alaska King, cooked, steamed	6 oz	165	3	0	0
Blue, canned	6 oz	168	2	0	0
Blue, cooked	6 oz	173	3	0	0
Blue, crab cakes	2 oz	93	5	1	0
Dungeness, cooked	6 oz	187	2	0	0
Surimi (imitation)	6 oz	162	1	0	0

Crawfish (Crayfish)
Farmed, steamed	6 oz	148	2	0	0
Wild, steamed	6 oz	139	2	0	0

Lobster
Northern, cooked	6 oz	167	1	0	0
Spiny, cooked	6 oz	243	3	1	0

Shrimp
Canned	6 oz	170	2	0	0
Cooked, steamed	6 oz	168	2	0	0
Cooked, fried	6 oz	411	21	4	0
Surimi (imitation)	6 oz	172	3	0	0
Mussel, Blue, cooked	6 oz	292	8	1	0

Oyster
Eastern, canned	6 oz	117	4	1	0
Eastern, cooked, battered & fried	6 oz	335	↑21	↑5	0
Eastern, farmed, cooked, dry heat	6 oz	134	4	1	0
Eastern, farmed, raw	6 oz	100	3	1	0
Eastern, wild, cooked, dry heat	6 oz	122	3	1	0
Eastern, wild, raw	6 oz	116	4	1	0
Pacific, cooked	6 oz	277	8	2	0
Pacific, raw	6 oz	138	4	1	0

Chol (mg)	Sod (mg)	Carb (g)	Fiber (g)	Sugar (g)	Prot (g)
↑114	193	9	0	0	43
↑104	↑619	18	0	0	24
↑114	190	9	0	0	43
↑90	↑1822	0	0	0	33
↑151	↑566	0	0	0	35
↑170	↑474	0	0	0	34
↑90	198	0	0	0	12
↑129	↑643	0	0	0	38
34	↑1430	26	1	11	13
↑233	165	0	0	0	30
↑226	160	0	0	0	29
↑122	↑646	0	0	0	35
↑153	386	0	0	0	45
↑428	↑1321	0	0	0	35
↑332	381	0	0	0	36
↑301	↑585	20	0	0	37
↑61	↑1198	16	0	0	21
↑95	↑627	13	0	0	40
↑94	190	0	0	0	12
↑138	↑709	20	0	0	15
↑65	277	0	0	0	12
42	303	0	0	0	9
↑83	415	0	0	0	14
↑90	359	0	0	0	12
↑170	360	0	0	0	32
↑85	180	0	0	0	16

The Meat and Bean Group

Item	Serving	Cal	Total Fat (g)	Sat Fat (g)	Trans Fat (g)
Scallop					
Cooked, battered & fried	6 oz	366	↑19	↑5	0
Cooked, steamed	6 oz	190	2	0	0
Squid					
Cooked, battered & fried	6 oz	298	↑13	3	na
Shellfish, Dishes					
Gorton's®					
Beer Battered, Tempura Shrimp	5	240	12	↑3.5	0
Jumbo Butterfly, Tempura Shrimp	5	250	11	3	0
Lemon Butter, Tempura Shrimp	4 oz	120	6	2	0 ᴾ
Popcorn Shrimp	20	240	12	↑3.5	0
Van de Kamp's®					
Beer Battered Shrimp	6	200	6	2	0
Butterfly Shrimp breaded	7	250	11	↑3.5	0 ᴾ
Popcorn Shrimp, breaded	20	260	11	↑4.5	0 ᴾ

Chol (mg)	Sod (mg)	Carb (g)	Fiber (g)	Sugar (g)	Prot (g)
↑104	↑789	0	0	0	31
↑90	450	0	0	0	39
↑442	↑520	13	0	0	31
40	↑670	25	0	2	7
55	430	27	0 [E]	4	11
↑65	↑740	8	0	1	8
55	↑630	24	0	2	8
↑90	↑750	22	1 [E]	1	14
↑65	↑540	27	1 [E]	3	12
↑80	↑750	30	2	3	11

The Meat and Bean Group

Eggs

Eggs are considered part of the USDA Food Pyramid Meat and Bean Group.

USDA Recommendations:

Go lean on protein.

KEEP IT SIMPLE

Eat a total of 5.5 ounces per day— from the entire Meat and Bean Group. *USDA recommended Daily Serving is based on a 2,000 calorie diet.*

Eggs are a good source of protein, vitamins and minerals. Eggs are ↑ **in cholesterol.**

One egg contains approximately 200mg of **cholesterol.**

Egg whites **do not contain cholesterol** and have **little to no fat** or **saturated fat.**

The recommended Daily Value for cholesterol is 300mg, for a 2,000 calorie *and* a 2,500 calorie diet.

EAT SMART. Use two egg whites and one egg yolk to reduce overall calories, fat and cholesterol. To add flavor without adding fat try using chives, peppers, mushrooms and other herbs or vegetables when preparing eggs. Another option, consider using an egg substitute. Egg substitutes are mostly egg whites—with food coloring.

Item	Serving	Cal	Total Fat (g)	Sat Fat (g)	Trans Fat (g)
EGGS					
Fresh, whole, raw, small	1	54	4	1	0
Fresh, whole, raw, medium	1	63	4	1	0
Fresh, whole, raw, large	1	72	5	2	0
Fried, large	1	90	7	2	na
Hard Boiled, large	1	78	5	2	0
Poached, large	1	71	5	2	0
Scrambled, large	1	102	7	2	na
Whites, fresh, raw, large	1	17	0	0	0
Yolk, fresh, raw, large	1	55	5	2	0
Duck					
Fresh, raw	1	130	10	3	0
Goose					
Fresh, raw	1	266	↑19	↑5	0
Quail					
Fresh, raw	1	14	1	0	0
Turkey					
Fresh, raw	1	135	9	3	0
Egg Substitute					
Egg Beaters®	¼ cup	30	0	0	0

Chol (mg)	Sod (mg)	Carb (g)	Fiber (g)	Sugar (g)	Prot (g)
↑161	53	0	0	0	5
↑186	62	0	0	0	6
↑212	70	0	0	0	6
↑210	94	0	0	0	6
↑212	62	1	0	0	6
↑211	147	0	0	0	6
↑215	171	1	0	0	7
0	55	0	0	0	4
↑210	8	1	0	0	3
↑619	102	1	0	1	9
↑1227	199	2	0	1	20
↑76	13	0	0	0	1
↑737	119	1	0	0	11
0	115	1	0	1	6

The Milk Group

All fluid milk products and many foods made from milk are considered part of the USDA Food Pyramid Milk Group; this includes **Milk, Yogurt** and **Cheese.**

USDA Recommendations:

Go low fat or fat free.

If you don't or can't consume milk, choose lactose-free products or other calcium sources.

KEEP IT SIMPLE

Eat a total of 3 cups per day. *USDA recommended Daily Serving is based on a 2,000 calorie diet.*

Dairy provides eight essential nutrients including phosphorus, potassium, protein, vitamins D, A and B12, riboflavin and niacin (niacin equivalents).

Animal derived products like milk, yogurt and cheese contain **cholesterol.**

Cheese is an excellent source of calcium. A 1½ ounce serving of natural cheese has the same amount of calcium as one cup of milk; however, cheese can be ↑ **in sodium and** ↑ **saturated fat.** Smaller servings are recommended.

Whole milk products are ↑ **in saturated fat,** a nutrient that needs to be limited. Fat free or reduced fat 2% milk are better choices.

Flavored milk and yogurt can be high in added sweeteners such as sugar, High Fructose Corn Syrup and Artificial Sweeteners.

EAT SMART. Choose low fat milk, yogurt and cheese more often. Compare different brands of cheese to reduce sodium. Pick plain yogurt over flavored yogurt more often. For added flavor, toss in your favorite fresh or frozen fruit.

MILK

Item	Serving	Cal	Total Fat (g)	Sat Fat (g)	Trans Fat (g)
Lactose Free					
Lactaid®					
Fat Free	1 cup	80	0	0	0
Reduced Fat 2%	1 cup	130	5	3	0
Low Fat 1%	1 cup	110	2.5	1.5	0
Land O' Lakes®					
Fat Free Dairy Ease®	1 cup	90	0	0	0
Reduced fat 2%, Dairy Ease®	1 cup	130	5	3	0
Whole, Dairy Ease®	1 cup	160	9	↑5	0
Low Fat (1%)					
Horizon®, Organic	1 cup	100	2.5	1.5	0
Land O' Lakes®	1 cup	100	2.5	1.5	0
Shamrock Farms®	1 cup	100	2.5	1.5	0
Stremick's Heritage®, Organic	1 cup	120	2.5	1.5	0
Non Fat (skim)					
Horizon®, Organic	1 cup	90	0	0	0
Land O' Lakes®	1 cup	90	0	0	0
Shamrock Farms®	1 cup	90	0	0	0
Stremick's Heritage®, Organic	1 cup	90	0	0	0
Reduced Fat (2%)					
Horizon®, Organic	1 cup	120	5	3	0
Land O' Lakes®	1 cup	120	5	3	0
Shamrock Farms®	1 cup	120	4.5	3	0
Stremick's Heritage®, Organic	1 cup	130	5	3	0
Whole					
Horizon®, Organic	1 cup	150	8	↑5	0
Land O' Lakes®	1 cup	150	8	↑5	0
Shamrock Farms®	1 cup	150	8	↑5	0
Stremick's Heritage®, Organic	1 cup	150	8	↑5	0

Chol (mg)	Sod (mg)	Carb (g)	Fiber (g)	Sugar (g)	Prot (g)
5	125	12	0	12	8
20	125	12	0	12	8
10	125	12	0	12	8
5	125	12	0	12	8
15	130	12	0	12	9
20	125	11	0	11	8
10	125	12	0	12	8
15	125	13	0	13	8
10	125	12	0	12	8
10	150	14	0	14	11
5	130	12	0	12	9
5	125	13	0	13	8
5	125	12	0	11	8
5	120	12	0	12	9
20	125	12	0	12	8
20	125	12	0	12	13
20	120	12	0	12	8
25	130	13	0	13	10
35	125	12	0	12	8
35	125	12	0	12	8
30	115	11	0	11	8
35	115	11	0	11	8

Item	Serving	Cal	Total Fat (g)	Sat Fat (g)	Trans Fat (g)
Flavored Milk					
Chocolate					
Hershey's®, Milk Shake, bottle	na	270	8	↑4.5	0
Hershey's®, Milk Shake, reduced fat, bottle	na	200	5	3	0
Hershey's®, Milk Shake, no sugar added, 1% low fat, bottle	na	120	2.5	2	0
Land O' Lakes®, Swiss Chocolate, 2% low fat, bottle	1 cup	190	5	3	0
Nesquik®, Milk Shake, bottle	1 cup	180	4	3	0
Nesquik®, reduced fat milk, bottle	1 cup	200	5	3	0
Shamrock® Mmmmilk, bottle	12 oz	340	↑13	↑8	0
Strawberry					
Hershey®, Milk Shake, bottle	na	280	7	↑4.5	0
Hershey®, Milk Shake, reduced fat, bottle	na	200	5	3	0
Nesquik®, reduced fat milk, bottle	1 cup	200	5	3	0
Shamrock® Mmmmilk reduced fat, bottle	12 oz	330	7	↑4.5	0

YOGURT

Item	Serving	Cal	Total Fat (g)	Sat Fat (g)	Trans Fat (g)
Dannon®					
Blueberries n' Cream, Light & Fit	4 oz	60	3	2	0
Blueberry, All Natural	3.3 oz	110	1	1	0
Blueberry, Fruit at the Bottom	6 oz	140	1.5	1	0
Cherry, Fruit at the Bottom	6 oz	140	1.5	1	0
Peach, All Natural	3.3 oz	110	1	1	0
Peach, Fruit Blend	6 oz	170	1.5	1	0
Peaches n' Cream, Light & Fit	4 oz	60	3	2	0
Plain, All Natural	4 oz	80	4	2.5	0
Strawberry & Banana, Fruit Blend	6 oz	160	1.5	1	0

Chol (mg)	Sod (mg)	Carb (g)	Fiber (g)	Sugar (g)	Prot (g)
20	140	43	1	41	10
20	135	31	1	28	8
5	170	15	1	13 [A]	11
20	220	26	0	26	8
10	120	29	1	28	8
15	150	32	1	30	8
50	300	44	1	31	14
20	220	44	0	44	9
15	130	30	0	29	8
15	120	33	0	31 [HF]	8
35	220	44	0	42 [HF]	15

10	25	3	0	2 [A]	5
5	65	20	0	19	5
5	130	26	1	25 [HF]	6
5	280	26	0	24 [HF]	6
5	65	20	0	19	5
10	125	33	0	30 [HF]	6
10	25	3	0	2 [A]	5
10	60	6	0	6	9
10	100	30	0	27 [HF]	6

The Milk Group

Item	Serving	Cal	Total Fat (g)	Sat Fat (g)	Trans Fat (g)
Stonyfield Farms®					
Blueberry, Organic, low fat	6 oz	130	1.5	↑5	0
French Vanilla, fat free	1 cup	180	0	0	0
French Vanilla, Organic	6 oz	190	6	↑4	0
Plain, fat free	1 cup	100	0	0	0
Strawberry & Cream, Organic	6 oz	170	6	↑3.5	0
Strawberry, fat free	1 cup	180	0	0	0
Strawberry, Organic, low fat	1 cup	220	2.5	1.5	0
Wallaby®					
Blueberry, Organic, low fat	6 oz	150	2.5	1.5	0
Plain, Organic, non fat	1 cup	130	0	0	0
Strawberry, Organic, low fat	6 oz	150	2.5	1.5	0
Strawberry, Organic, non fat	6 oz	140	0	0	0
Vanilla, Organic, low fat	6 oz	150	2.5	1.5	0
Vanilla Bean, Organic, non fat	6 oz	140	0	0	0
Yoplait®					
Blueberry, light	6 oz	100	0	0	0
Chocolate Mousse, Whips®	4 oz	160	4	2.5	0
French Vanilla	6 oz	170	1.5	1	0
Strawberry	6 oz	170	1.5	1	0
Strawberry, light	6 oz	100	0	0	0
Yogurt Drinks					
Dannon®					
Berries n' Cream, Light & Fit, Smoothie	7 oz	60	2.5	1.5	0
Peach Passion, Light & Fit, Smoothie	7 oz	60	0	0	0
Plain, DanActive®	3.3 oz	90	1.5	1.5	0
Strawberry, DanActive®	3.3 oz	90	1.5	1.5	1
Stonyfield Farms®					
Peach, Smoothie, All Natural	10 oz	250	3	2	0

Chol (mg)	Sod (mg)	Carb (g)	Fiber (g)	Sugar (g)	Prot (g)
5	95	25	2	22	6
0	140	36	3	33	9
25	95	27	3	24	6
0	150	18	3	15	10
20	90	24	2	22	5
0	150	36	3	32	9
10	135	42	4	36	9
15	75	26	0	20	7
15	150	19	0	10	12
15	75	26	0	21	7
10	90	27	0	20	7
15	75	25	0	20	6
10	90	28	0	22	7
5	85	19	0	14 [HF, A]	5
15	105	25	0	22 [HF]	5
10	80	33	0	27 [HF]	5
0	80	33	0	27 [HF]	5
5	85	19	0	14 [HF,A]	5
15	35	4	0	3 [A]	6
5	85	9	0	6 [A]	5
5	40	15	0	15	3
5	45	17	0	17	3
10	150	49	4	44	10

The Milk Group

Item	Serving	Cal	Total Fat (g)	Sat Fat (g)	Trans Fat (g)
Yogurt Drinks continued					
Stonyfield Farms®					
Strawberry, Smoothie, Organic, light	10 oz	130	0	0	0
Vanilla, Smoothie, All Natural	10 oz	250	3	2	0
Wild Berry, Smoothie, Organic, light	10 oz	130	0	0	0
Kefir					
Lifeway®					
Peach, Smoothie, Organic, low fat	1 cup	110	2.5	1.5	0
Plain, Smoothie, Organic	1 cup	160	8	⬆5	0
Plain, Smoothie, Organic, low fat	1 cup	110	2.5	1.5	0
Plain, Smoothie, Slim 6®, low carb	1 cup	110	2	1.5	0
Strawberry & Banana, Smoothie, Slim 6®, low carb	1 cup	110	2	1.5	0
Strawberry n' Crème, Smoothie, Organic	1 cup	160	8	⬆5	0

CHEESE

Item	Serving	Cal	Total Fat (g)	Sat Fat (g)	Trans Fat (g)
Blue					
Crumbles	1 oz	95	8	⬆5	0
Lighthouse®, Idaho Bleu Cheese, crumbles	¼ cup	100	8	⬆5	0
Rosenborg®, Danish Blue Cheese, crumbles	1 oz	100	8	⬆5	0
Wedge	1 oz	100	8	⬆5	0
Brick					
Shredded	1 oz	84	7	⬆4	0
Wedge	1 oz	105	8	⬆5	0
Brie	1 oz	95	8	⬆5	0
Camembert	1 oz	85	7	⬆4	0
Caraway	1 oz	107	8	⬆5	0
Cheddar					
Cello®, sliced	1 oz	110	9	⬆5	0
Boar's Head®, Sharp, deli	1 oz	110	9	⬆5	0

Chol (mg)	Sod (mg)	Carb (g)	Fiber (g)	Sugar (g)	Prot (g)
0	90	41	3	19	9
10	150	46	4	41	10
0	90	41	3	19	9
10	125	12	3	8	14
30	125	12	3	8	10
10	125	12	3	8	14
10	125	8	2	6 [A]	14
10	125	8	2	6 [A]	14
30	125	12	3	8	10

20	377	1	0	0	6
35	400	2	0	0	5
15	310	0	0	0	6
21	395	1	0	0	6
21	127	1	0	0	5
27	159	1	0	0	7
28	178	0	0	0	6
20	239	0	0	0	6
26	196	1	0	0	7
30	180	1	0	0	7
30	190	1	0	0	7

The Milk Group

Item	Serving	Cal	Total Fat (g)	Sat Fat (g)	Trans Fat (g)
Cheddar continued					
Horizon®					
Organic, Cheddar, bar	1 oz	110	9	↑5	0
Organic, Cheddar, finely shredded	¼ cup	110	9	↑5	0
Organic, Cheddar, slice	1 oz	80	7	↑4	0
Sharp, Organic, bar	1 oz	110	9	↑5	0
Kraft®					
Fat Free, Cheddar, shredded	1 oz	45	0	0	0
Medium Cheddar, block	1 oz	120	10	↑6	0
Mild, Natural, 2% low fat, bar	1 oz	90	6	↑4	0
Mild, 2% low fat, shredded	1 oz	80	6	↑3.5	0
Mild, shredded	¼ cup	110	9	↑6	0
Sharp, Deluxe, 2% low fat, sliced	1 slice	70	5	3	0
Sharp, 2% low fat, bar	1 oz	90	6	↑4	0
Cheddar, Sargento®, Sharp, sliced	1 slice	80	6	↑4	0
Cheshire	1 oz	110	9	↑6	0
Colby					
Boar's Head®, Colby Jack, deli	1 oz	110	9	↑6	0
Sargento®, sliced	1 oz	80	7	↑4	0
Cottage Cheese					
Creamed	½ cup	116	5	3	0
Low Fat, 1%	½ cup	81	1	1	0
Low Fat, 2%	½ cup	102	2	1	0
Edam, Boar's Head®, deli	1 oz	90	7	↑5	0
Feta					
Athenos®, reduced fat, crumbles	¼ cup	70	4.5	3	0
Crumbles	¼ cup	99	8	↑6	0
Fontina	1 oz	110	9	↑5	0
Goat					
Hard	1 oz	128	10	↑7	0
Soft	1 oz	76	6	↑4	0

Cheese

Chol (mg)	Sod (mg)	Carb (g)	Fiber (g)	Sugar (g)	Prot (g)
30	180	1	0	0	7
30	180	1	0	0	7
20	135	0	0	0	5
30	180	1	0	0	7
5	280	1	0	0	9
30	180	0	0	0	6
20	240	1	0	0	7
20	230	1	0	0	7
25	190	1	0	0	6
15	190	1	0	0	6
20	240	1	0	0	7
20	140	0	0	0	5
29	198	1	0	0	7
25	180	0	0	0	6
20	140	1	0	0	5
17	458	3	0	0	14
5	459	3	0	3	14
9	459	4	0	0	16
20	280	0	0	0	7
10	↑470	1	1	0	7
33	418	2	0	2	5
33	227	0	0	0	7
30	98	1	0	1	9
13	104	0	0	0	5

The Milk Group | 163

Item	Serving	Cal	Total Fat (g)	Sat Fat (g)	Trans Fat (g)
Cheese continued					
Gorgonzola Salemville®, Amish, rBST free, crumbles	1 oz	100	8	↑5	0
Gouda					
Boar's Head®, deli	1 oz	110	9	↑5	0
Cello®, sliced	1 oz	110	9	↑5	0
Gruyere	1 oz	117	9	↑5	0
Havarti					
Boar's Head®, Dill, Plain or Jalapeno	1 oz	110	10	↑7	0
Cello®, sliced	1 oz	110	9	↑6	0
Limburger	1 oz	93	8	↑5	0
Monterey Jack					
Boar's Head®, deli	1 oz	100	9	↑6	0
Horizon®, Organic, finely shredded	¼ cup	100	8	↑4.5	0
Sargento®, Monterey Jack, sliced	1 slice	80	6	↑4	0
Mozzarella					
Horizon®, Organic, shredded	¼ cup	80	5	3	0
Horizon®, Organic, String Cheese	1	80	5	3	0
Kraft®, shredded, 2% low fat	¼ cup	70	4	2.5	0
Kraft®, String Cheese, 2% low fat	1	70	4	2.5	0
Sargento®, sliced	1 slice	60	4	2.5	0
Muenster					
Alpine Lace®, sliced	1 slice	100	9	↑5	0
Boar's Head®, deli	1 oz	100	8	↑5	0
Sargento®, sliced	1	80	6	↑4	0
Neufchatel	1 oz	74	7	1	0
Parmesan					
Grated	1 oz	122	8	↑5	0
Grated, Kraft®	2 tbsp	25	1.5	1	0
Hard	1 oz	111	7	↑5	0
Low sodium	1 oz	128	8	↑5	0
Shredded	1 oz	116	8	↑5	0

Chol (mg)	Sod (mg)	Carb (g)	Fiber (g)	Sugar (g)	Prot (g)
25	260	0	0	0	7
30	280	0	0	0	6
25	270	1	0	0	7
31	95	0	0	0	8
35	210	0	0	0	6
25	170	1	0	0	6
26	227	0	0	0	6
25	180	0	0	0	6
30	170	0	0	0	7
20	135	0	0	0	5
15	170	1	0	0	8
1	170	1	0	0	8
15	200	1	0	0	8
15	220	1	0	0	8
10	140	1	0	0	5
20	85	0	0	0	7
20	75	0	0	0	6
20	135	0	0	0	5
22	113	1	0	0	3
25	433	1	0	0	11
5	100	0	0	0	2
19	454	1	0	0	10
22	18	1	0	0	12
20	↑475	1	0	0	11

The Milk Group

Item	Serving	Cal	Total Fat (g)	Sat Fat (g)	Trans Fat (g)
Parmesan *continued*					
Shredded, Horizon®, Organic, finely shredded	1 tbsp	20	1.5	1	0
Provolone					
Boar's Head®, deli	1 oz	100	8	↑4.5	0
Sargento®, reduced fat, sliced	1	50	3.5	2	0
Ricotta					
Part skim milk	½ cup	171	10	↑6	0
Whole milk	½ cup	216	↑16	↑10	0
Romano	1 oz	110	8	↑5	0
Roquefort	1 oz	105	9	↑5	0
Swiss					
Cello®, sliced	1 oz	120	9	↑6	0
Finlandia®, Light Swiss, sliced	1 slice	57	3	2	0
Kraft®, Natural, 2% low fat, sliced	1 slice	70	4.5	3	0
Kraft®, Deli Deluxe, thin slice	1 slice	110	9	↑5	0
Sargento®, Deli Style, thin slice	1 slice	70	5	3	0
Sargento®, reduced fat, sliced	1	60	4	2	0

Chol (mg)	Sod (mg)	Carb (g)	Fiber (g)	Sugar (g)	Prot (g)
5	70	0	0	0	2
20	140	1	0	0	7
10	140	0	0	0	5
38	155	6	0	0	14
↑63	104	4	0	0	14
29	340	1	0	0	9
26	↑513	1	0	0	6
25	50	0	0	0	8
8	110	0	0	0	7
15	50	0	0	0	6
30	50	0	0	0	8
20	40	0	0	0	5
10	30	1	0	0	7

Oils

Oils are fats which are liquid at room temperature. Oils come from plant foods and from fish.

USDA Recommendations:

Eat all fat sparingly.

KEEP IT SIMPLE

Eat six teaspoons of oil or less per day. *USDA recommended Daily Serving is based on a 2,000 calorie diet.*

Plant oils are ↑ **in unsaturated fat** (monounsaturated and polyunsaturated fats) and **low in saturated fat,** which is good. An exception is tropical oils, such as coconut and palm oil.

Take a moment to look at the list of oils found in the Oils chapter. Look at the "Total Fat" column. Notice, the entire column lists "14" grams of fat for every type of oil. Now look at the "Sat Fat" (saturated fat) column, "Tropical" oils are the only oils ↑ **in saturated fat.** These oils should be used less often.

Plant oils **do not contain cholesterol.**

Fish, nut and vegetable oils **do not raise** "bad" **cholesterol** blood levels and therefore are good substitutes for butter, lard or shortening.

As a general rule, oils from plants are extracted chemically. Cold Pressed or Expeller Pressed oils are extracted naturally without chemicals.

Most oils are refined to withstand high heat. The refining process includes bleaching and deodorizing the extracted oil. Unrefined oils don't go through this process. They have a richer color and retain most of their nutritional properties. Unrefined oils are labeled as "unrefined." Most are not suitable for high heat cooking.

EAT SMART. Choose oils with two grams or less of saturated fat. Watch your overall consumption. Many foods are naturally high in oil including nuts, olives, avocados and fish.

Item	Serving	Cal	Total Fat (g)	Sat Fat (g)	Trans Fat (g)
OILS					
Almond	1 tbsp	120	↑14	1	0
Apricot Kernel	1 tbsp	120	↑14	1	0
Avocado, Spectrum®	1 tbsp	120	↑14	2	0
Canola					
Crisco®	1 tbsp	120	↑14	1	0
Spectrum®, Organic, refined	1 tbsp	120	↑14	1	0
Spectrum®, High Heat, refined	1 tbsp	120	↑14	1	0
Wesson®	1 tbsp	120	↑14	1	0
Corn					
Crisco®	1 tbsp	120	↑14	2	0
Spectrum®, unrefined	1 tbsp	120	↑14	2	0
Wesson®	1 tbsp	120	↑14	2	0
Flaxseed	1 tbsp	120	↑14	1	0
Fish Oils					
Cod Liver	1 tbsp	123	↑14	3	0
Salmon	1 tbsp	123	↑14	3	0
Grapeseed	1 tbsp	120	↑14	1	0
Olive					
Extra Virgin, Crisco®	1 tbsp	120	↑14	2	0
Extra Virgin, Spectrum®, Organic	1 tbsp	120	↑14	2	0
Extra Virgin, Spectrum®, Organic, unrefined	1 tbsp	120	↑14	2	0
Light, Crisco®	1 tbsp	120	↑14	2	0
Pure, Crisco®	1 tbsp	120	↑14	2	0
Peanut					
Crisco®	1 tbsp	120	↑14	2.5	0
Spectrum®, unrefined	1 tbsp	120	↑14	3	0
Safflower					
Spectrum®, Organic, refined	1 tbsp	120	↑14	1	0
Spectrum®, unrefined	1 tbsp	120	↑14	1	0
Sunflower					
High Oleic	1 tbsp	124	↑14	1	0

Chol (mg)	Sod (mg)	Carb (g)	Fiber (g)	Sugar (g)	Prot (g)
0	0	0	0	0	0
0	0	0	0	0	0
0	0	0	0	0	0
0	0	0	0	0	0
0	0	0	0	0	0
0	0	0	0	0	0
0	0	0	0	0	0
0	0	0	0	0	0
0	0	0	0	0	0
0	0	0	0	0	0
0	0	0	0	0	0
↑78	0	0	0	0	0
↑66	0	0	0	0	0
0	0	0	0	0	0
0	0	0	0	0	0
0	0	0	0	0	0
0	0	0	0	0	0
0	0	0	0	0	0
0	0	0	0	0	0
0	0	0	0	0	0
0	0	0	0	0	0
0	0	0	0	0	0
0	0	0	0	0	0
0	0	0	0	0	0

Oils

Item	Serving	Cal	Total Fat (g)	Sat Fat (g)	Trans Fat (g)
Sunflower continued					
Linoleic	1 tbsp	120	↑14	1	0
Sesame, Spectrum®, Organic, unrefined	1 tbsp	120	↑14	2	0
Soy, Spectrum®, Organic, refined	1 tbsp	120	↑14	2	0
Tropical					
Coconut, Spectrum®, Organic, refined	1 tbsp	120	↑14	↑12	0
Coconut, Spectrum®, Organic unrefined	1 tbsp	120	↑14	↑12	0
Palm Oil	1 tbsp	120	↑14	↑7	0
Palm Kernel Oil	1 tbsp	117	↑14	↑11	0
Vegetable (soybean), Crisco®	1 tbsp	120	↑14	2	0
Walnut	1 tbsp	120	↑14	2	0

Chol (mg)	Sod (mg)	Carb (g)	Fiber (g)	Sugar (g)	Prot (g)
0	0	0	0	0	0
0	0	0	0	0	0
0	0	0	0	0	0
0	0	0	0	0	0
0	0	0	0	0	0
0	0	0	0	0	0
0	0	0	0	0	0
0	0	0	0	0	0

Discretionary or Optional Choices

"Discretionary or Optional Choices," covers a variety of food not necessarily part of the five main food groups. As a result, the following chapters will not provide Daily Serving recommendations:

Dairy and Non Dairy

Butter, Lard, Margarine and Shortening

Condiments, Salad Dressing and Mayonnaise

Herbs, Spices, Salt and Seasonings

Sauces, Gravies, Marinades

Jelly, James, Sweeteners and Syrup

Soup

Each chapter will offer valuable tips on best choices and ways to EAT SMART.

EAT SMART. Opt for low fat foods and products low in added sugar from this group. Watch for foods/products labeled as "fat free" because they may still contain Trans Fats (partially hydrogenated oils).

Dairy and Non-Dairy

Diary foods low in calcium and/or high in fat, and Non Dairy products are *not* part of the USDA Food Pyramid Milk Group. This includes **Butter, Buttermilk, Cream, Cream Cheese** and **Sour Cream, Non Dairy Creamers, Rice** and **Soy milk,** and **yogurts.**

Dairy provides eight essential nutrients, including phosphorus, potassium, protein, vitamins D, A and B12, riboflavin and niacin (niacin equivalents).

Butter, buttermilk, cream, cream cheese and sour cream are dairy products considered discretionary choices and should be eaten in moderation, as should any food ⬆ **in fat.**

Animal derived products, such as dairy, contain **cholesterol.**

Non Dairy calcium fortified foods and beverages, such as soy products, are a healthy option for vegetarians (those who only eat foods of plant origin) and for those who are lactose intolerant.

Non Dairy creamers, including fat free creamers labeled "0 Trans Fat per serving," may still contain **Trans Fats**—the worst kind of fat. These products are coded with a [P].

Please locate the "Non Dairy" section in this chapter and then go to "Creamers." Notice, the "Trans Fat" column lists "0" for all creamers, but the first brand's creamers are coded with a [P] meaning these products contain Trans

Fats. The serving size is 1 tbsp (one tablespoon). This is good news if you only use one tablespoon. If not, you may want to consider another brand that doesn't contain Partially Hydrogenated Oils (Trans Fat). Trans Fats can quickly add up.

EAT SMART. Choose low fat or fat free dairy. If you choose whole milk or other full fat dairy products, balance your meal with other low fat foods.

DAIRY

Item	Serving	Cal	Total Fat (g)	Sat Fat (g)	Trans Fat (g)
Buttermilk					
Low Fat	1 cup	98	2	1	0
Reduced Fat	1 cup	137	5	3	0
Condensed Milk					
Carnation®, sweetened	2 tbsp	130	3	2	0
Eagle Brand®, sweetened	2 tbsp	130	3	2	0
Eagle Brand®, fat free	2 tbsp	110	0	0	0
Santini®, Organic, sweetened	2 tbsp	130	3	2	0
Cream					
Half and Half	2 tbsp	39	3	2	0
Half and Half	1 cup	315	↑28	↑17	0
Half and Half, fat free	2 tbsp	18	0	0	0
Half and Half, fat free	1 cup	132	3	2	0
Heavy, fluid cream, whipped	1 cup	414	↑44	↑28	0
Reddi-wip®, original	2 tbsp	15	1	.5	0
Cream Cheese					
Chive & Onion, Philadelphia®, light	2 tbsp	60	4.5	3	0
Strawberry, Philadelphia®, light	2 tbsp	70	4	2.5	0
Plain, Horizon®, Organic	2 tbsp	110	10	↑6	0
Plain, Horizon®, Organic, reduced fat	2 tbsp	70	7	↑4	0
Plain, Philadelphia®	2 tbsp	90	9	↑5	0
Plain, Philadelphia®, block	1 oz	100	9	↑6	0
Plain, Philadelphia®, light	2 tbsp	60	4.5	3	0
Plain, Philadelphia®, fat free, block	1 oz	30	0	0	0
Whipped, Philadelphia®	2 tbsp	60	6	↑3.5	0
Cheese Product					
Cheez Whiz, Cheese Sauce	2 tbsp	90	7	1.5	0
Kraft®, American, Singles	1 slice	70	5	3	0

Chol (mg)	Sod (mg)	Carb (g)	Fiber (g)	Sugar (g)	Prot (g)
10	257	12	0	12	8
20	211	13	0	13	10
10	45	22	0	22	3
10	40	23	0	23	3
5	40	24	0	24	3
10	40	23	0	23	3
11	12	1	0	0	1
↑90	99	11	0	0	7
2	43	3	0	1.5	1
11	323	20	0	11	6
↑164	46	3	0	0	2
5	0	1	0	1	0
15	170	2	0	2	3
15	120	6	0	5	2
30	90	1	0	0	2
25	100	2	0	1	2
35	130	2	0	2	2
40	105	1	0	1	2
15	150	2	0	2	3
5	200	2	0	1	4
20	90	1	0	1	1
5	440	4	0	2	3
20	270	2	0	1	4

Discretionary or Optional Choices

Item	Serving	Cal	Total Fat (g)	Sat Fat (g)	Trans Fat (g)
Cheese Product *continued*					
Kraft®, American, 2% low fat, Singles	1 slice	50	2.5	1.5	0
Evaporated Milk					
Carnation®	2 tbsp	40	2	1.5	0
Carnation®, fat free	2 tbsp	25	0	0	0
Sour Cream	2 tbsp	51	5	3	0
Sour Cream, reduced fat	2 tbsp	40	4	3	0
Velveeta	1 oz	80	6	↑3.5	0
Whipped Topping, Cool Whip®	2 tbsp	25	1.5	1.5	0 [H]

NON-DAIRY

Item	Serving	Cal	Total Fat (g)	Sat Fat (g)	Trans Fat (g)
Creamer					
Coffee-mate®					
Hazelnut, fluid	1 tbsp	35	1.5	0	0 [P]
Hazelnut, fluid, fat free	1 tbsp	25	0	0	0 [P]
Hazelnut, fluid, sugar free	1 tbsp	15	1	0	0 [P]
Irish Crème, fluid	1 tbsp	35	0	0	0 [P]
Original, fluid	1 tbsp	20	1	0	0 [P]
Original, fluid, single serving	1 creamer	15	1.5	1	0
Original, powder	1 tsp	10	.5	.5	0 [P]
International Delight®					
French Vanilla, fat free	1 tbsp	30	0	0	0
Hazelnut, fluid	1 tbsp	45	2	1	0
Hazelnut, fluid, sugar free	1 tbsp	20	2	1	0
Hazelnut, fluid, single serving	1 creamer	40	2	1	0
Irish Cream, fluid	1 tbsp	40	1.5	1	0
Southern Pecan, fluid	1 tbsp	40	1.5	1	0
Rice Milk					
Rice Dream®, Original, refrigerated	1 cup	120	2.5	0	0
Rice Dream®, Vanilla, refrigerated	1 cup	130	2.5	0	0

Dairy and Non Dairy

Chol (mg)	Sod (mg)	Carb (g)	Fiber (g)	Sugar (g)	Prot (g)
10	290	2	0	2	4
10	30	3	0	3	2
0	40	4	0	4	2
11	13	1	0	0	1
12	12	1	0	0	1
20	410	3	0	2	5
0	0	2	0	1 [HF]	0

0	10	5	0	5 [HF]	0
0	0	5	0	4	0
0	5	1	0	0 [A]	0
0	10	5	0	5	0
0	0	2	0	1	0
0	0	0	0	0	0
0	0	1	0	0	0
5	0	7	0	6	0
0	5	6	0	5	0
0	0	1	0	0 [A]	0
0	5	5	0	5	0
0	0	7	0	6	0
0	10	7	0	6	0
0	80	23	0	10	1
0	80	26	0	12	1

Discretionary or Optional Choices

Item	Serving	Cal	Total Fat (g)	Sat Fat (g)	Trans Fat (g)
Soy Milk					
Silk®					
Chocolate, refrigerated	1 cup	140	3.5	.5	0
Plain, refrigerated	1 cup	100	4	.5	0
Plain, refrigerated, light	1 cup	70	2	0	0
Very Vanilla, refrigerated	1 cup	130	4	.5	0
Soy Dream®, Original, Organic, refrigerated	1 cup	100	3.5	.5	0
Soy Yogurt					
Blueberry, O'Soy, Stonyfield Farm®	6 oz	170	2	0	0
Chocolate, O'Soy, Stonyfield Farm®	6 oz	160	3	0	0
Vanilla, O'Soy, Stonyfield Farm®	6 oz	150	2	0	0

Chol (mg)	Sod (mg)	Carb (g)	Fiber (g)	Sugar (g)	Prot (g)
0	100	23	2	19	5
0	120	8	1	6	7
0	120	8	1	6	16
0	140	19	1	16	16
0	140	9	2	5	8
0	35	33	4	27	7
0	30	28	4	22	7
0	40	26	4	21	7

Butter, Lard, Margarine and Shortening

Butter, Lard, stick **Margarine** and **Shortening** are considered solid fats. Solid fats are fats solid at room temperature.

Solid fats are found in many animal derived foods including butter, beef, chicken and pork (lard) fat. In addition, animal products, such as these, contain **cholesterol.**

Hydrogenation is the chemical process used to turn vegetable oils into a solid fat, i.e. stick margarine and shortening.

Solid fats (foods/products with hydrogenated fat or animal derived fats) are ↑ **in saturated fats.** Saturated fats, also known as artery clogging fats, should be limited.

Trans Fats (partially hydrogenated oil), another harmful fat, can be found in shortening, stick margarine and even "heart healthy" tub margarines labeled "0 Trans Fat per serving." Products containing Partially Hydrogenated Oil are coded with a [P] in this chapter.

Diets high in saturated fat and/or Trans Fat are risk factors for many diseases. The Daily Value for saturated fat is less than 20 grams, based on a 2,000 calorie diet. A guideline for Trans Fat is less than two grams per day. Zero is best.

EAT SMART. Use liquid oils with two grams or less of saturated fat (see the Oils chapter) instead of solid fats—Butter, Lard and Shortening. Tub Margarines are available with no Trans Fats and are a good option for a buttery spread. Check the INGREDIENTS list for "partially hydrogenated" oil and avoid Trans Fats.

BUTTER, LARD, MARGARINE and SHORTENING

Item	Serving	Cal	Total Fat (g)	Sat Fat (g)	Trans Fat (g)
Butter					
Salted	1 tbsp	102	12	↑7	0
Salted, whipped	1 tbsp	67	8	↑5	0
without salt	1 tbsp	102	12	↑7	0
Beef Fat (tallow, suet)	1 tbsp	115	↑13	↑13	0
Chicken Fat	1 tbsp	115	↑13	↑4	0
Lard (pork fat)	1 tbsp	115	↑13	↑5	0
Margarine					
Benecol®, soft spread	1 tbsp	70	8	1	0 [P]
Benecol®, soft spread light	1 tbsp	50	5	.5	0 [P]
Brummel & Brown®, soft spread	1 tbsp	45	5	1	0 [P]
Fleischmann's®					
Soft spread, made with olive oil	1 tbsp	70	8	1.5	0 [P]
Soft spread, original	1 tbsp	70	8	1.5	0 [P]
Soft spread, unsalted	1 tbsp	70	8	1.5	0 [P]
I Can't Believe It's Not Butter®					
Soft spread	1 tbsp	80	8	2	0 [P]
Soft spread, light	1 tbsp	50	5	1	0 [P]
Stick	1 tbsp	90	10	2	2.5 [P]
Stick, light	1 tbsp	50	6	1	1.5 [P]
Parkay®					
Soft spread	1 tbsp	60	7	1.5	0 [P]
Soft spread, light	1 tbsp	50	5	1	na [P]
Stick	1 tbsp	80	9	2	0 [P]
Stick, light	1 tbsp	50	5	1	na [P]
Promise®, soft spread	1 tbsp	80	8	1.5	0
Promise®, soft spread, light	1 tbsp	45	5	1	0
Smart Balance® soft spread	1 tbsp	80	9	2.5	0
Smart Balance®, soft spread, light	1 tbsp	45	5	1.5	0
Take Control®, soft spread	1 tbsp	80	8	1	0
Take Control®, soft spread light	1 tbsp	45	5	1	0

Chol (mg)	Sod (mg)	Carb (g)	Fiber (g)	Sugar (g)	Prot (g)
31	82	0	0	0	0
21	78	0	0	0	0
31	2	0	0	0	0
14	0	0	0	0	0
11	0	0	0	0	0
12	0	0	0	0	0
0	110	0	0	0	0
0	110	0	0	0	0
0	90	0	0	0	0
0	95	0	0	0	0
0	75	0	0	0	0
0	0	0	0	0	0
0	90	0	0	0	0
0	85	0	0	0	0
0	95	0	0	0	0
0	85	0	0	0	0
0	100	0	0	0	0
0	130	0	0	0	0
0	110	0	0	0	0
0	75	0	0	0	0
0	85	0	0	0	0
0	85	0	0	0	0
0	90	0	0	0	0
0	85	0	0	0	0
5	85	0	0	0	0
5	85	0	0	0	0

Item	Serving	Cal	Total Fat (g)	Sat Fat (g)	Trans Fat (g)
Shortening					
Fully Hydrogenated	1 tbsp	113	↑13	3	0 [H]
Hydrogenated & Partially hydrogenated	1 tbsp	113	↑13	3	4 [H,P]
Crisco®, Zero Trans Fat	1 tbsp	106	12	3	0 [H,P]

Chol (mg)	Sod (mg)	Carb (g)	Fiber (g)	Sugar (g)	Prot (g)
0	0	0	0	0	0
0	0	0	0	0	0
0	0	0	0	0	0

Condiments, Salad Dressing and Mayonnaise

Condiments, Salad Dressings and **Mayonnaise** are used to accompany or flavor food.

Condiments such as pickles, relish, ketchup and mustard are **fat free** and can be ↑ **in sodium** or contain added sweeteners.

Salad Dressing and Mayonnaise may be ↑ **in fat.** In fact, one serving (two tablespoons) of Salad Dressing can be higher in fat than a six ounce steak.

If you enjoy ↑ fat Salad Dressing, consider limiting the high fat extras such as nuts and cheese to balance out total fat.

Trans Fats (partially hydrogenated oil) and **cholesterol** are found in some cream based dressings and mayonnaise.

EAT SMART. Low fat and low sodium varieties of Condiments, Salad Dressings and Mayonnaise are available, select these products more often. Carefully review the INGREDIENTS list for products with Partially Hydrogenated Oil and avoid Trans Fats. Compare NUTRITION FACTS on like products in this guide and on grocery store shelves.

Item	Serving	Cal	Total Fat (g)	Sat Fat (g)	Trans Fat (g)
CONDIMENTS					
Capers, canned	1 tbsp	2	0	0	0
Chili Sauce, Dynasty®	1 tsp	10	1	0	0
Cocktail Sauce					
Heinz®, Seafood Cocktail	¼ cup	60	0	0	0
Kraft®, original	¼ cup	60	.5	0	0
Zatarain's®, original	¼ cup	70	0	0	0
Hoisin Sauce	1 tbsp	35	1	0	0
Horseradish					
Creamed, Inglehoffer®	1 tsp	10	.5	0	0
Creamed, Beaver®, hot	1 tsp	10	.5	0	0
Prepared, Beaver®, extra hot	1 tsp	5	0	0	0
Ketchup					
Annie's Naturals®, Organic	1 tbsp	15	0	0	0
Heinz® original	1 tbsp	15	0	0	0
Heinz®, original, Organic	1 tbsp	20	0	0	0
Heinz®, reduced sugar	1 tbsp	5	0	0	0
Hunts®, original	1 tbsp	15	0	0	0
Hunts®, no salt	1 tbsp	20	0	0	0
Muir Glenn®, Organic	1 tbsp	20	0	0	0
Mustard					
Annie's Naturals®					
Dijon Mustard, Organic	1 tsp	0	0	0	0
Honey Mustard, Organic	1 tsp	10	0	0	0
Horseradish Mustard, Organic	1 tsp	5	0	0	0
Yellow, Organic	1 tsp	0	0	0	0
French's®, Classic Yellow	1 tsp	0	0	0	0
French's®, Spicy Brown	1 tsp	5	0	0	0
Grey Poupon®					
Country Dijon	1 tsp	5	0	0	0
Dijon	1 tsp	5	0	0	0
Harvest Ground	1 tsp	45	0	0	0
Hebrew National®, Kosher	1 tsp	4	0	0	0

Chol (mg)	Sod (mg)	Carb (g)	Fiber (g)	Sugar (g)	Prot (g)
0	255	0	0	0	0
0	80	1	0	0	0
0	↑690	15	1	11 HF	0
0	↑880	11	0	9	1
0	↑950	17	0	13	1
0	258	7	0	4	1
0	20	1	0	0 HF	0
0	20	1	0	0 HF	0
0	35	1	0	0 HF	0
0	150	3	0	2	0
0	190	4	0	4 HF	0
0	190	5	0	4	0
0	190	1	0	1 A	0
0	180	4	0	4 HF	0
0	0	4	0	4 HF	0
0	230	4	0	3	0
0	120	0	0	0	0
0	40	2	0	2	0
0	90	1	0	1	0
0	55	0	0	0	0
0	55	0	0	0	0
0	80	0	0	0	0
0	120	0	0	0	0
0	120	0	0	0	0
0	120	0	0	0	0
0	65	0	0	0	0

Discretionary or Optional Choices

Item	Serving	Cal	Total Fat (g)	Sat Fat (g)	Trans Fat (g)
Mustard *continued*					
Inglehoffer®, Stone ground	1 tsp	10	0	0	0
Plochman's®, Yellow	1 tsp	0	0	0	0
Plochman's®, Natural Stone Ground	1 tsp	5	0	0	0
Zatarain's®, Creole Mustard	1 tsp	10	.5	0	0
Olives					
Calamata, Mezzetta®, pitted, jar	4	40	4	0	0
Green Manzanillo, Early California®, Pimento stuffed, jar	4	25	2	0	0
Black, Early California®, pitted, medium, canned	5	25	2.5	0	0
Orange Sauce					
Iron Chef®	2 tbsp	60	0	0	0
Lee Kum Kee®	2 ½ tbsp	80	0	0	0
Pickles					
Back to Nature®, Kosher Dill, Wholes, refrigerated	½ pickle	5	0	0	0
Claussen®, Hearty Garlic, Sandwich slices, refrigerated	2	5	0	0	0
Vlassic®					
Bread & Butter, stackers	1	30	0	0	0
Dill, Hamburger Style, oval chips	3 slices	25	0	0	0
Kosher Dill, spears	¾ spear	5	0	0	0
Polish Dill, spears	¾ spear	5	0	0	0
Relish, Dill	1 tbsp	5	0	0	0
Relish, Sweet	1 tbsp	15	0	0	0
Soy Sauce					
Kikkoman®, original	1 tbsp	10	0	0	0
Kikkoman, less sodium	1 tbsp	10	0	0	0
La Choy®, original	1 tbsp	10	0	0	0
La Choy®, lite sodium	1 tbsp	15	0	0	0

Chol (mg)	Sod (mg)	Carb (g)	Fiber (g)	Sugar (g)	Prot (g)
0	75	1	1	0	0
0	5	0	0	0	0
0	60	0	0	0	0
0	150	1	0	0	0
0	240	1	0	0	0
0	330	1	0	0	0
0	115	1	0	0	0
0	100	15	0	13	0
0	50	19	0	15	0
0	330	1	0	0	0
0	320	1	0	1	0
0	170	7	0	6 [HF]	0
0	390	1	0	1 [HF]	0
0	210	1	0	1	0
0	280	1	0	1	0
0	240	1	0	1	0
0	140	4	0	4 [HF]	0
0	↑920	0	0	0	2
0	↑575	1	0	0	1
0	↑1160	1	0	1	1
0	↑550	2	0	2	1

Discretionary or Optional Choices

Item	Serving	Cal	Total Fat (g)	Sat Fat (g)	Trans Fat (g)
Sauerkraut					
Canned	1 oz	5	0	0	0
Canned, low sodium	1 oz	6	0	0	0
Hebrew National®, Kosher, refrigerated	2 tbsp	5	0	0	0
Salsa					
Amy's®, Medium, Organic	2 tbsp	10	0	0	0
Amy's®, Spicy Chipotle, Organic	2 tbsp	10	0	0	0
La Victoria®, Ranchera, hot	2 tbsp	10	0	0	0
La Victoria®, Salsa Verge, medium	2 tbsp	10	0	0	0
La Victoria®, Thick & Chunky, mild	2 tbsp	10	0	0	0
Muir Glen®, Black Bean & Corn, Organic	2 tbsp	20	0	0	0
Muir Glen®, Medium, Organic	2 tbsp	10	0	0	0
Ortega®, Smokey Chipotle, medium	2 tbsp	10	0	0	0
Ortega®, Thick & Chunky, medium	2 tbsp	10	0	0	0
Pace Picante®, hot	2 tbsp	10	0	0	0
Pace Picante®, Organic, medium	2 tbsp	10	0	0	0
Pace Picante®, mild	2 tbsp	10	0	0	0
Steak Sauce					
A1®, Kobe Sesame Teriyaki	1 tbsp	15	0	0	0
A1®, Cracked Peppercorn	1 tbsp	15	0	0	0
A1®, original	1 tbsp	15	0	0	0
Heinz 57®, original	1 tbsp	20	0	0	0
Newman's Own®	1 tbsp	20	0	0	0
Sweet & Sour Sauce					
Kikkoman's®, original	2 tbsp	30	0	0	0
La Choy®, original	2 tbsp	60	0	0	0
World Harbor®, Maui Mountain	2 tbsp	60	0	0	0

Chol (mg)	Sod (mg)	Carb (g)	Fiber (g)	Sugar (g)	Prot (g)
0	185	1	1	1	0
0	86	1	1	0	0
0	180	1	1	0	0
0	190	2	0	1	0
0	160	2	0	1	0
0	160	2	0	1	0
0	140	2	0	1	0
0	200	2	0	1	0
0	135	4	1	1	1
0	130	3	0	1	0
0	210	2	1	1	0
0	190	3	0	1	0
0	230	2	1	2	0
0	250	2	1	2	0
0	250	2	1	2	0
0	280	3	0	2	0
0	260	2	1	2	0
0	280	3	0	2	0
0	190	4	0	4 [HF]	0
0	85	4	0	1	0
0	190	9	0	7	0
0	110	14	0	11	0
0	250	14	0	12 [HF]	0

Item	Serving	Cal	Total Fat (g)	Sat Fat (g)	Trans Fat (g)
Taco Sauce					
Green, La Victoria®, mild	1 tbsp	5	0	0	0
Red, Ortega®, mild	1 tbsp	10	0	0	0
Red, La Victoria, medium	1 tbsp	5	0	0	0
Tartar Sauce					
Beaver®, Seafood Tartar Sauce	2 tbsp	16	2.5	0	0
Best Foods®	2 tbsp	80	7	1	0
Kraft®	2 tbsp	60	4.5	.5	0
Tobasco					
Green Pepper	1 tsp	0	0	0	0
Habanera	1 tsp	5	0	0	0
Original	1 tsp	0	0	0	0
Worcestershire					
Lea & Perrins®	1 tsp	5	0	0	0
The Wizards®, Organic, Vegan	1 tsp	0	0	0	0

SALAD DRESSING – Creamy

Item	Serving	Cal	Total Fat (g)	Sat Fat (g)	Trans Fat (g)
Blue Cheese					
Kraft®, Blue Cheese	2 tbsp	120	⬆13	2	0
Wishbone®, Chunky Blue Cheese	2 tbsp	150	⬆15	2.5	0 [P]
Wishbone®, fat free	2 tbsp	35	0	0	0 [P]
Buttermilk					
Annie's Naturals®, Organic	2 tbsp	70	7	1	0
Hidden Valley®, Buttermilk	2 tbsp	140	⬆14	2	0
Catalina, Kraft®	2 tbsp	100	6	1	0
Caesar					
Annie's Naturals®, Organic	2 tbsp	120	12	1.5	0
Kraft® Caesar	2 tbsp	110	11	2	0 [P]
Kraft®, free	2 tbsp	50	0	0	0
Newman's Own®, Organic	2 tbsp	170	⬆18	2	0
Wishbone®, Creamy Caesar	2 tbsp	170	⬆18	3	0

Chol (mg)	Sod (mg)	Carb (g)	Fiber (g)	Sugar (g)	Prot (g)
0	70	1	0	0	0
0	120	2	0	1	0
0	90	1	0	1	0
15	160	1	0	1 HF	0
19	320	5	0	3	0
5	230	4	0	3 HF	0
0	140	0	0	0	0
0	140	1	0	1	0
0	30	0	0	0	0
0	65	1	0	1 HF	0
0	120	1	0	1	0

5	290	1	0	1	0
5	260	2	0	1 HF	0
0	280	7	1	3	1
10	210	1	0	1	1
10	340	2	0	1	0
0	420	10	0	9 HF	0
5	170	1	0	1	1
5	310	1	0	0	1
0	310	1	0	0	1
13	330	1	0	0	0
10	330	1	0	1	1

Discretionary or Optional Choices

Item	Serving	Cal	Total Fat (g)	Sat Fat (g)	Trans Fat (g)
Ceasar *continued*					
Wishbone®, Creamy Caesar, light	2 tbsp	50	2	.5	0
French					
Annie's Naturals®, Organic	2 tbsp	90	9	.5	0
Wishbone®, Deluxe	2 tbsp	120	11	1.5	0
Goddess, Annie's Naturals®	2 tbsp	120	↑13	1	0
Honey Mustard					
Wishbone®, Honey Dijon, light	2 tbsp	50	2	0	0
Italian					
Newman's Own®, Creamy Italian	2 tbsp	140	↑14	2.5	0
Wishbone®, Creamy Italian	2 tbsp	110	10	1.5	0
Wishbone®, Country Italian, light	2 tbsp	30	1.5	0	0
Ranch					
Hidden Valley®					
Bacon Ranch	2 tbsp	140	↑14	2.5	0
Fat Free	2 tbsp	30	0	0	0
Light	2 tbsp	80	7	1	0
Original	2 tbsp	140	↑14	2.5	0
Original, Organic	2 tbsp	140	↑14	2	0
Spicy Ranch	2 tbsp	150	↑16	2	0
Kraft®					
Cucumber Ranch	2 tbsp	110	11	1.5	0
Light	2 tbsp	70	4.5	.5	0
Original	2 tbsp	110	11	1.5	0
Peppercorn Ranch	2 tbsp	110	11	2	0
Newman's Own®, original Ranch	2 tbsp	140	↑15	2	0
Wishbone®, original	2 tbsp	160	↑13	2	0
Wishbone®, Carb Options, Ranch	2 tbsp	150	↑17	2.5	0
Wishbone®, light, Ranch	2 tbsp	40	2	0	0

Chol (mg)	Sod (mg)	Carb (g)	Fiber (g)	Sugar (g)	Prot (g)
10	310	7	0	2	1
5	170	3	0	3	0
0	170	5	0	5 HF	0
0	250	1	0	1	0
0	250	8	1	6 HF	0
10	270	2	0	1	1
0	240	4	0	2 HF	0
0	330	3	0	2	0
0	230	1	0	1	1
0	310	6	0	3	0
5	290	3	0	2	1
10	260	2	0	1	1
10	220	2	0	1	1
10	320	2	0	1	0
0	210	3	0	2	0
10	370	7	0	1	0
5	310	2	0	1	0
0	270	2	0	1	0
10	250	2	0	2	0
5	250	2	0	2 HF	0
10	210	0	0	0 A	0
0	290	5	0	2	0

Discretionary or Optional Choices

Item	Serving	Cal	Total Fat (g)	Sat Fat (g)	Trans Fat (g)
Thousand Islands					
Annie's Naturals®, Organic	2 tbsp	90	7	1	0
Kraft®, original	2 tbsp	80	6	1	0
Newman's Own®	2 tbsp	140	⬆14	2	0
Wishbone®, original	2 tbsp	130	12	2	0
Wishbone, light	2 tbsp	50	2	0	0

SALAD DRESSING – Oil and Vinaigrettes

Item	Serving	Cal	Total Fat (g)	Sat Fat (g)	Trans Fat (g)
Balsamic					
Annie's Naturals®, Organic, Vinaigrette	2 tbsp	100	10	.5	0
Kraft®, Vinaigrette, light	2 tbsp	25	1	0	0
Kraft®, Vinaigrette, original	2 tbsp	90	8	1	0
Newman's Own® original	2 tbsp	90	9	1	0
Newman's Own®, Lighten Up!	2 tbsp	45	4	0	0
Wishbone®, Vinaigrette	2 tbsp	50	5	.5	0
Wishbone®, Balsamic Breeze, Salad Spritzers™	10 sprays	10	1	0	0
Caesar					
Girard's® light	2 tbsp	90	8	1.5	0
Girard's®, original	2 tbsp	140	⬆15	2.5	0
Newman's Own®, Lighten Up!	2 tbsp	70	6	1	0
Newman's Own®, original	2 tbsp	150	⬆16	1.5	0
Wishbone®, original	2 tbsp	170	⬆18	3	0
Wishbone®, Caesar Delight, Salad Spritzers™	10 sprays	15	1	0	0
Honey Mustard, Annie's Naturals®, Vinaigrette, low fat	2 tbsp	45	2	0	0
Italian					
Girard's®, original	2 tbsp	130	⬆13	2	0
Kraft®, Zesty Italian, fat free	2 tbsp	15	0	0	0
Newman's Own®, Family Recipe	2 tbsp	120	⬆13	1	0

Salad Dressings

Chol (mg)	Sod (mg)	Carb (g)	Fiber (g)	Sugar (g)	Prot (g)
5	140	5	0	4	1
5	330	6	0	5 ᴴᶠ	0
10	260	4	0	3	0
10	330	5	0	4 ᴴᶠ	0
5	290	9	0	0 ᴴᶠ	0

0	75	3	0	3	0
0	290	4	0	3	0
0	300	4	0	3	0
0	350	3	0	1	0
0	270	2	0	1	0
0	280	3	0	3 ᴴᶠ	0
0	130	1	0	1 ᴴᶠ	0
10	370	5	0	2	1
10	360	1	0	1	1
5	↑520	3	0	2	1
0	420	1	0	1	1
10	300	1	0	1	1
0	85	1	0	1 ᴴᶠ	0
0	200	6	0	6	0
0	↑510	2	0	1	0
0	↑480	3	0	2 ᴴᶠ	0
0	400	1	0	1	1

Discretionary or Optional Choices

Item	Serving	Cal	Total Fat (g)	Sat Fat (g)	Trans Fat (g)
Italian *continued*					
Newman's Own®, Lighten Up!	2 tbsp	60	6	1	0
Newman's Own®, Organic, Tuscan Italian	2 tbsp	100	11	1.5	0
Wishbone®, original	2 tbsp	90	8	1	0
Wishbone®, fat free	2 tbsp	20	0	0	0
Raspberry					
Annie's Naturals®, Vinaigrette	2 tbsp	35	1.5	0	0
Girard's®, Vinaigrette, fat free	2 tbsp	60	0	0	0
Kraft®, Vinaigrette, light	2 tbsp	60	4	0	0
Newman's Own®, Raspberry & Walnut, Lighten Up!	2 tbsp	70	5	.5	0
Red Wine, Wishbone®, Vinaigrette, fat free	2 tbsp	30	0	0	0

MAYONNAISE

Item	Serving	Cal	Total Fat (g)	Sat Fat (g)	Trans Fat (g)
Best Foods®, original	1 tbsp	90	10	1.5	0
Best Foods, light	1 tbsp	40	4.5	.5	0
Dynasty®, Thai Hot Chili	1 tbsp	110	12	1	0
Dynasty®, Wasabi	1 tbsp	100	11	2	0
Kraft®, original	1 tbsp	90	10	1.5	0
Kraft®, light	1 tbsp	50	5	.5	0
Miracle Whip®, original	1 tbsp	40	3	0	0
Miracle Whip®, light	1 tbsp	20	1.5	0	0
Spectrum®, Artisan Dijon	1 tbsp	90	10	1.5	0
Spectrum®, Artisan Wasabi	1 tbsp	100	11	2	0
Spectrum®, Canola Mayonnaise	1 tbsp	100	11	.5	0
Spectrum®, Eggless, Vegan, Light Canola	1 tbsp	35	3.5	0	0
Spectrum®, Organic	1 tbsp	100	11	2	0

Chol (mg)	Sod (mg)	Carb (g)	Fiber (g)	Sugar (g)	Prot (g)
0	260	0	0	0	0
0	380	1	0	1	0
0	↑490	3	0	3 HF	0
0	350	4	0	3 HF	0
0	75	5	0	4	0
0	210	14	0	11 HF	0
0	270	5	0	5	0
0	120	7	0	5	0
0	230	7	0	6 HF	0

5	90	0	0	0	0
5	115	1	0	0	0
10	80	0	0	0	0
10	70	0	0	0	0
5	70	0	0	0	0
5	95	1	0	1	0
5	125	2	0	2 HF	0
5	135	2	0	1 HF	0
10	90	1	0	0	0
10	65	0	0	0	0
5	90	0	0	0	0
0	65	0	0	0	0
10	65	0	0	0	0

Discretionary or Optional Choices

Herbs, Spices, Salt and Seasonings

Herbs, Spices, Salt and **Seasonings** are used to flavor food.

Herbs and Spices are naturally **fat free** and **low sodium.**

Seasonings can be blends of herbs and/or salts.

Salt based seasonings are generally ↑ **in sodium** and may contain **Trans Fats** (partially hydrogenated oil).

The recommended Daily Value for sodium is less than 2,400mg, based on a 2,000 calorie diet.

¼ of a teaspoon of salt is typically 590mg of sodium—or 25% of the recommended Daily Value.

Compare products such as salt—yes, salt—with other salts. Amazingly enough, the sodium content varies and it's one of the easiest ways to reduce sodium. Take a moment to look up "Salt' in this chapter, go to "white" salt and notice two brands of salt that can save you 200mg to 260 mg per serving.

Sodium is essential for nerves, muscles and for maintaining the electrolyte balance inside and outside of cells. In excess, sodium may be harmful to your health. Check with your doctor or health care provider before making dietary changes.

EAT SMART. To reduce sodium, season foods with herbs, spices or salt free blends. Read the INGREDIENTS list on all products and pass up products with Partially Hydrogenated Oils (Trans Fats).

HERBS, SPICES, SALT and SEASONINGS

Item	Serving	Cal	Total Fat (g)	Sat Fat (g)	Trans Fat (g)
Herbs and Spices					
Allspice, ground	1 tsp	5	0	0	0
Anise seed	1 tsp	7	0	0	0
Basil, dried	1 tsp	4	0	0	0
Basil, fresh	1 tbsp	1	0	0	0
Bay Leaf	1 tsp	2	0	0	0
Caraway Seed	1 tsp	7	0	0	0
Cardamom	1 tsp	6	0	0	0
Celery Seed	1 tsp	8	1	0	0
Chili Powder	1 tsp	8	0	0	0
Cinnamon, ground	1 tsp	6	0	0	0
Cloves, ground	1 tsp	7	0	0	0
Cilantro (coriander)	1 tsp	2	0	0	0
Cumin Seed	1 tsp	8	0	0	0
Curry Powder	1 tsp	6	0	0	0
Dill Weed, dried	1 tsp	3	0	0	0
Dill Weed, fresh	10 sprigs	1	0	0	0
Fennel Seed	1 tsp	7	0	0	0
Garlic Powder	1 tsp	9	0	0	0
Ginger Root, fresh	1 tsp	2	0	0	0
Ginger, ground	1 tsp	6	0	0	0
Marjoram, dried	1 tsp	2	0	0	0
Nutmeg	1 tsp	12	1	0	0
Onion Powder	1 tsp	8	0	0	0
Oregano, dried	1 tsp	6	0	0	0
Paprika	1 tsp	6	0	0	0
Parsley	1 tsp	1	0	0	0
Parsley, fresh	1 tbsp	1	0	0	0
Pepper, Black	1 tsp	5	0	0	0
Pepper, Red (cayenne)	1 tsp	6	0	0	0
Rosemary, dried	1 tsp	4	0	0	0
Rosemary, fresh	1 tbsp	2	0	0	0
Sage	1 tsp	2	0	0	0
Tarragon. dried	1 tsp	5	0	0	0
Turmeric, ground	1 tsp	8	0	0	0

Chol (mg)	Sod (mg)	Carb (g)	Fiber (g)	Sugar (g)	Prot (g)
0	1	1	0	0	0
0	0	1	0	0	0
0	0	1	0	0	0
0	0	0	0	0	0
0	0	0	0	0	0
0	0	1	0	0	0
0	0	1	0	0	0
0	3	1	0	0	0
0	26	1	0	0	0
0	1	2	0	0	0
0	5	1	0	0	0
0	1	0	0	0	0
0	4	1	0	0	0
0	1	1	0	0	0
0	2	1	0	0	0
0	1	0	0	0	0
0	2	1	0	0	0
0	1	2	0	0	0
0	0	0	0	0	0
0	1	1	0	0	0
0	0	0	0	0	0
0	0	1	0	1	0
0	1	2	0	1	0
0	0	1	1	0	0
0	1	1	1	0	0
0	2	0	0	0	0
0	2	0	0	0	0
0	1	1	0	0	0
0	1	1	0	0	0
0	0	1	0	0	0
0	0	0	0	0	0
0	0	0	0	0	0
0	1	1	0	0	0
0	1	1	0	0	0

Discretionary or Optional Choices

Item	Serving	Cal	Total Fat (g)	Sat Fat (g)	Trans Fat (g)
Salt					
Grey, Celtic Sea Salt®, fine ground	¼ tsp	0	0	0	0
Grey, Celtic®, light	¼ tsp	0	0	0	0
Pink, Himalayan Pink®, Jurassic Salt	¼ tsp	0	0	0	0
Red, Alaea®, Hawaiian Sea Salt	¼ tsp	0	0	0	0
White					
Bob's Red Mill®, Premium Sea Salt	¼ tsp	0	0	0	0
Hain®, Sea Salt	¼ tsp	0	0	0	0
Lima®, Atlantic Sea Salt	¼ tsp	0	0	0	0
Morton®, Iodized	¼ tsp	0	0	0	0
Redmond®, Gourmet Kosher Sea Salt	¼ tsp	0	0	0	0
Seasonings					
Emeril's®, Chicken Rub	¼ tsp	0	0	0	0
Emeril's®, Rib Rub	¼ tsp	0	0	0	0
Lawry's®					
Chili Seasoning, packet	1 tsp	10	0	0	0
Garlic Salt	¼ tsp	0	0	0	0
Lemon Pepper	¼ tsp	0	0	0	0
Taco Seasoning, packet	2 tsp	15	0	0	0
Salt Free 17	¼ tsp	0	0	0	0
Sloppy Joes Seasoning, packet	2 tsp	20	0	0	0
Season Salt	¼ tsp	0	0	0	0
McCormick®					
Chili Seasoning, packet	1 tbsp	30	.5	0	0
Chili Seasoning, 30% less sodium, Packet	1 tbsp	30	.5	0	0
Garlic Herb Seasoning Blend	¼ tsp	0	0	0	0 [P]
Roasted Garlic & Bell Pepper Blend	¼ tsp	10	0	0	0
Rub, Chicken	2 tsp	15	0	0	0
Rub, Pork	2 tsp	15	0	0	0
Rub, Seafood	2 tsp	15	0	0	0 [P]
Rub, Steak	2 tsp	15	0	0	0 [P]

Chol (mg)	Sod (mg)	Carb (g)	Fiber (g)	Sugar (g)	Prot (g)
0	330	0	0	0	0
0	410	0	0	0	0
0	↑580	0	0	0	0
0	↑580	0	0	0	0
0	390	0	0	0	0
0	↑590	0	0	0	0
0	330	0	0	0	0
0	↑590	0	0	0	0
0	↑530	0	0	0	0
0	80	0	0	0	0
0	160	0	0	0	0
0	↑500	2	0	0	0
0	240	0	0	0	0
0	80	0	0	0	0
0	340	3	1	0	0
0	0	0	0	0	0
0	↑480	5	0	3	0
0	380	0	0	0	0
0	310	5	0	0	1
0	210	5	0	0	1
0	50	0	0	0	0
0	370	2	0	0	0
0	260	2	0	1	0
0	220	2	0	1	0
0	190	3	0	1	0
0	440	2	0	1	0

Discretionary or Optional Choices

Item	Serving	Cal	Total Fat (g)	Sat Fat (g)	Trans Fat (g)
Seasonings continued					
Sloppy Joes Seasoning, packet	1 tsp	20	0	0	0
Taco, mild seasoning, packet	2 tsp	20	0	0	0
Mrs. Dash®					
Chicken, Grill Blend, salt free	¼ tsp	0	0	0	0
Lemon Pepper, salt free	¼ tsp	0	0	0	0
Original, salt free	¼ tsp	0	0	0	0
Steak, Grill Blend, salt free	¼ tsp	0	0	0	0
Molly Mc Butter®					
Butter Flavor Sprinkles	1 tsp	5	0	0	0 [P]
Cheese Flavor Sprinkles	1 tsp	5	0	0	0 [P]
Old Bay®					
Blackened Seasoning	½ tsp	0	0	0	0
Crab Cake Classic Seasoning, packet	1 tbsp	30	1	0	0
Rub, Seafood	¾ tsp	5	0	0	0
Seafood Seasoning	¼ tsp	0	0	0	0
Simply Organic®					
Sloppy Joe Seasoning, packet	1 ½ tsp	15	0	0	0
Southwest Taco Seasoning, packet	2 tsp	15	0	0	0
The Spice Hunter®					
Barbeque Grill Spice, salt free	¼ tsp	0	0	0	0
Cajun Creole Seasoning, salt free	¼ tsp	0	0	0	0
California Garlic Salt	¼ tsp	0	0	0	0
Mexican Seasoning, salt free	¼ tsp	0	0	0	0

Chol (mg)	Sod (mg)	Carb (g)	Fiber (g)	Sugar (g)	Prot (g)
0	300	3	0	0	0
0	460	4	0	0	1
0	0	0	0	0	0
0	0	0	0	0	0
0	0	0	0	0	0
0	0	0	0	0	0
0	180	1	0	0	0
0	125	1	0	0	0
0	95	0	0	0	0
30	290	2	0	0	0
0	210	0	0	0	0
0	160	0	0	0	0
0	320	3	0	0	0
0	380	4	1	0	1
0	0	0	0	0	0
0	0	0	0	0	0
0	290	0	0	0	0
0	0	0	0	0	0

Sauces, Gravies and Marinades

Sauces, Gravies and **Marinades** are used to top off or flavor pastas, meat, poultry or seafood.

Most sauces, gravies and marinades are ↑ **in sodium.**

Barbeque sauces and marinades are usually **low fat and cholesterol free,** ↑ **in sodium** and may contain added sweeteners such as High Fructose Corn Syrup.

Many cream based pasta sauces contain cholesterol and are ↑ **in fat and** ↑ **saturated fat.**

Pasta sauce made from tomatoes range from **high fat to low fat** depending on the type of sauce. If meat is added, small amounts of **cholesterol** will be present.

EAT SMART. Choose low fat products to flavor food more often and occasionally treat yourself to higher fat creamy sauces; balance is key. To reduce sodium, compare similar or like products in this guide or at the grocery store. Consider low sodium sauces, gravies and marinades.

SAUCES

Item	Serving	Cal	Total Fat (g)	Sat Fat (g)	Trans Fat (g)
Alfredo					
Bertolli®, original, jar	¼ cup	110	10	↑5	0
Classico®, Creamy, jar	¼ cup	100	9	↑5	0
Ragu®, Classic, jar	¼ cup	110	10	3.5	0
Barbecue					
Annie's Naturals, original, Organic	2 tbsp	45	1	0	0
Annie's Naturals, Smokey Maple, Organic	2 tbsp	45	1	0	0
Bill Johnson's®, BBQ, original	2 tbsp	40	0	0	0
Bill Johnson's®, Hickory	2 tbsp	40	0	0	0
Jack Daniels®, Hickory Brown Sugar	2 tbsp	50	0	0	0
Jack Daniels®, Honey Smokehouse	2 tbsp	50	0	0	0
Jack Daniels®, Original #7	2 tbsp	50	0	0	0
Kraft®, Hickory Smoke	2 tbsp	50	0	0	0
Kraft®, Mesquite Smoke	2 tbsp	40	0	0	0
Kraft®, original	2 tbsp	50	0	0	0
Buffalo Wing Sauce					
Budweiser®	2 tbsp	25	1.5	0	0
Texas Pete's®, Buffalo Style Chicken Wing Sauce	2 tbsp	30	1	0	0
Orange Sauce					
Iron Chef®	2 tbsp	60	0	0	0
Lee Kum Kee®	2 ½ tbsp	80	0	0	0
Pasta Sauces					
Amy's®, Garlic Mushroom, Organic	½ cup	120	7	2.5	0
Amy's®, Family Marinara, Organic	½ cup	80	3	.5	0
Ragu®, Traditional	½ cup	70	2.5	0	0
Ragu®, Flavored with Meat	½ cup	70	3	.5	0
Muir Glen®, Cabernet Marinara, Organic	½ cup	60	0	0	0
Muir Glen®, Four Cheese, Organic	½ cup	60	1	0	0

Chol (mg)	Sod (mg)	Carb (g)	Fiber (g)	Sugar (g)	Prot (g)
40	460	3	0	1	2
50	410	3	0	1	2
30	400	3	0	2	1
0	240	9	0	5	0
0	220	9	0	5	0
0	260	10	0	9	0
0	260	10	0	9	0
0	290	13	0	10 HF	0
0	290	12	0	11 HF	0
0	290	12	0	8 HF	0
0	430	12	0	10 HF	0
0	420	9	0	7 HF	0
0	440	12	0	10 HF	0
0	↑730	3	0	1	0
0	↑830	5	2	0	1
0	100	15	0	13	0
0	50	19	0	15	0
5	↑680	10	3	5	3
0	↑590	10	3	5	1
0	↑580	9	2	6	2
0	↑570	9	2	6	2
0	360	11	2	4	2
0	370	12	2	4	2

Discretionary or Optional Choices | 217

Item	Serving	Cal	Total Fat (g)	Sat Fat (g)	Trans Fat (g)
Pasta Sauces *continued*					
Newman's Own®					
Five Cheese	½ cup	80	3	1.5	0
Marinara	½ cup	70	2	0	0
Tomato Basil, Organic	½ cup	90	4	.5	0
Traditional Herb, Organic	½ cup	90	4	.5	0
Prego®					
Italian Sausage & Garlic	½ cup	120	5	1.5	0
Marinara	½ cup	100	5	1	0
Tomato & Basil, Organic	½ cup	90	2.5	0	0
Progresso®					
Lobster, Pasta Sauce	½ cup	100	7	1	0
Red Clam, Pasta Sauce	½ cup	60	1	0	0
White Clam, Pasta Sauce	½ cup	130	10	1.5	0
Peanut Sauce, House of Tsang®	1 tbsp	45	2.5	0 [H]	0
Pesto, Classico®	¼ cup	230	21	3	0 [P]
Soy Sauce					
Kikkoman®, original	1 tbsp	10	0	0	0
Kikkoman, less sodium	1 tbsp	10	0	0	0
La Choy®, original	1 tbsp	10	0	0	0
La Choy®, lite sodium	1 tbsp	15	0	0	0
Sweet & Sour Sauce					
Kikkoman's®, original	2 tbsp	30	0	0	0
La Choy®, original	2 tbsp	60	0	0	0
World Harbor®, Maui Mountain	2 tbsp	60	0	0	0

GRAVY and MARINADES

Gravy					
Au jus, canned	½ cup	19	0	0	0
Beef, canned	½ cup	61	3	0	0
Chicken, canned	½ cup	94	7	0	0
Mushroom, canned	½ cup	60	3	0	0
Turkey, canned	½ cup	61	3	0	0

Chol (mg)	Sod (mg)	Carb (g)	Fiber (g)	Sugar (g)	Prot (g)
5	↑610	10	1	0	3
0	↑510	12	1	11	2
0	↑650	12	1	11	2
0	↑660	13	1	12	2
10	↑500	16	3	10	3
0	↑550	11	4	7	2
0	↑540	15	4	11	2
5	430	6	2	3	3
10	350	8	1	4	4
0	↑750	5	0	1	6
0	240	4	0	3	1
0	↑720	6	1	2	3
0	↑920	0	0	0	2
0	↑575	1	0	0	1
0	↑1160	1	0	1	1
0	↑550	2	0	2	1
0	190	9	0	7	0
0	110	14	0	11	0
0	250	14	0	12 [HF]	0

0	60	3	0	0	1
0	↑653	6	1	0	5
0	↑687	7	1	0	3
0	↑679	7	1	0	2
0	↑687	6	1	0	3

Discretionary or Optional Choices

Item	Serving	Cal	Total Fat (g)	Sat Fat (g)	Trans Fat (g)
Marinades					
Annie's Naturals®, Steak Marinade, Organic	2 tbsp	50	3.5	.5	0
Annie's Naturals®, Spicy Ginger Marinade, Organic	2 tbsp	35	2	0	0
A1®, Classic	1 tbsp	15	0	0	0
A1®, New Orleans Cajun	1 tbsp	25	0	0	0
KA·ME, Thai Coconut	1 tbsp	40	4	.5	0
KC Masterpiece®, Caribbean Jerk	1 tbsp	25	0	0	0
KC Masterpiece®, Steakhouse	1 tbsp	40	1.5	0	0
Lawry's®, Baja Chipotle	1 tbsp	15	0	0	0
Lawry's®, Louisiana Red Pepper	1 tbsp	10	0	0	0
Lawry's ®, Mesquite	1 tbsp	5	0	0	0
Newman's Own®, Lemon Pepper	1 tbsp	15	0	0	0
Teriyaki					
KC Masterpiece®, Ginger Teriyaki	1 tbsp	30	.5	0	0
Kikkoman's®, original	1 tbsp	15	0	0	0
Kikkoman's®, less sodium	1 tbsp	15	0	0	0
Lawry's®, original	1 tbsp	20	0	0	0
Newman's Own®, original	1 tbsp	25	0	0	0
Soy Vay®, Island Teriyaki	1 tbsp	30	.5	0	0
Soy Vay®, Veri Veri Teriyaki	1 tbsp	35	1	0	0
World Harbor®, Maui Mountain Teriyaki	2 tbsp	70	0	0	0

Chol (mg)	Sod (mg)	Carb (g)	Fiber (g)	Sugar (g)	Prot (g)
0	↑470	5	0	4	1
0	450	3	0	2	1
0	290	4	0	2 HF	0
0	180	5	0	5 HF	0
0	195	2	0	0	0
0	320	6	0	5 HF	0
0	310	7	0	6 HF	0
0	320	4	0	2 HF	0
0	390	2	0	1 HF	0
0	350	1	0	0 HF	0
0	300	3	0	2	0
0	360	8	0	7 HF	0
0	↑610	2	0	2 HF	1
0	320	3	0	3	1
0	↑560	4	0	4 HF	0
0	330	6	0	4	0
0	320	5	0	4	1
0	↑490	6	0	5	0
0	270	17	0	15 HF	0

Jelly, Jams, Sweeteners and Syrup

Jelly and Jams are used as spreads. **Sweeteners,** caloric and non caloric, are used to sweeten a variety of foods. **Syrups** are popular for topping pancakes and desserts.

Jelly and jams, sweeteners and syrups **do not contain fat, saturated fat or cholesterol.** Most contain High Fructose Corn Syrup. An exception being Organic jams and spreads. Organic products as a whole do not contain High Fructose Syrup and are a good option.

Artificial Sweeteners are low in calories and do not affect blood sugar levels; however, certain foods (such as carbohydrates) containing Artificial Sweeteners can.

Natural Sweeteners such as stevia and agave nectar have a low Glycemic rating (effect on blood glucose level) and are considered safe for diabetics. Please check with your health care provider before making changes to your diet.

Many pancake and flavored syrups are made with High Fructose Corn Syrup. Pure maple syrups are all natural and do not contain High Fructose Corn Syrup or added sodium.

EAT SMART. To reduce added sweeteners consider low sugar or "no sugar added" jams and jellies or pure all natural syrups. Natural or Artificial Sweeteners are a matter of personal choice.

Item	Serving	Cal	Total Fat (g)	Sat Fat (g)	Trans Fat (g)
JELLY and JAMS					
Apple Butter, Smucker's®, Spiced	1 tbsp	45	0	0	0
Apricot					
Cascadian Farms®, Organic, Spread	1 tbsp	40	0	0	0
Smucker's®, Preserves, low sugar	1 tbsp	25	0	0	0
Blackberry					
Cascadian Farms®, Organic, Spread	1 tbsp	40	0	0	0
Smucker's®, Jam	1 tbsp	50	0	0	0
Smucker's®, Jelly	1 tbsp	50	0	0	0
Blueberry					
Cascadian Farms®, Organic, Spread	1 tbsp	40	0	0	0
Smucker's®, Preserves	1 tbsp	50	0	0	0
Cherry, Smucker's®, Preserves	1 tbsp	50	0	0	0
Fig Preserves, Braswell®	1 tbsp	45	0	0	0
Grape					
Cascadian Farms®, Organic, Spread	1 tbsp	40	0	0	0
Smucker's®, Concord Grape, Jam	1 tbsp	50	0	0	0
Smucker's®, Concord Grape, Jelly	1 tbsp	50	0	0	0
Smucker's®, Concord Grape, sugar free	1 tbsp	10	0	0	0
Welch's®, Concord Grape, Jam	1 tbsp	50	0	0	0
Welch's®, Concord Grape, Jelly	1 tbsp	50	0	0	0
Guava, Smucker's®, Jelly	1 tbsp	50	0	0	0
Pear Preserves, Braswell®	1 tbsp	50	0	0	0
Pepper					
Dickinson®, Cherry Pepper, Spread	1 tbsp	50	0	0	0
Dickinson®, Hot Pepper, Spread	1 tbsp	50	0	0	0
Orange Marmalade					
Smucker's®, low sugar	1 tbsp	25	0	0	0

Chol (mg)	Sod (mg)	Carb (g)	Fiber (g)	Sugar (g)	Prot (g)
0	10	11	0	10	0
0	0	10	0	10	0
0	0	6	0	5	0
0	0	10	0	10	0
0	0	13	0	12 HF	0
0	0	13	0	12 HF	0
0	0	10	0	10	0
0	0	13	0	12 HF	0
0	0	13	0	12 HF	0
0	0	11	0	9 HF	0
0	0	10	0	10	0
0	0	13	0	12 HF	0
0	5	13	0	12 HF	0
0	0	5	0	0 A	0
0	10	13	0	13 HF	0
0	15	13	0	13 HF	0
0	0	13	0	12 HF	0
0	10	14	0	12 HF	0
0	5	12	0	8	0
0	5	12	0	8	0
0	0	6	0	5	0

Discretionary or Optional Choices

Item	Serving	Cal	Total Fat (g)	Sat Fat (g)	Trans Fat (g)
Strawberry					
Cascadian Farms®, Organic, Spread	1 tbsp	40	0	0	0
Smucker's®, Jam	1 tbsp	50	0	0	0
Smucker's®, Jelly	1 tbsp	50	0	0	0
Smucker's®, sugar free	1 tbsp	10	0	0	0
Welch's®, Preserve	1 tbsp	50	0	0	0
Welch's®, Spread	1 tbsp	50	0	0	0

SUGAR and SWEETENERS

Sugar					
Brown					
C&H®, Dark Brown	1 tsp	15	0	0	0
C&H®, Golden Brown	1 tsp	15	0	0	0
Wholesome®, Organic, light	1 tsp	15	0	0	0
Powdered					
C&H®	¼ cup	120	0	0	0
Hain®, Organic	¼ cup	140	0	0	0
Raw					
Naturally Blond®, Sugar in the Raw	1 tsp	15	0	0	0
White					
C&H®, Pure Cane	1 tsp	15	0	0	0
C&H®, Pure Cane, Organic	1 tsp	15	0	0	0
Hain®, Organic	1 tsp	10	0	0	0
Sweeteners					
Agave Nectar, Sweet Cactus Farms®, Syrup, low glycemic	1 tsp	15	0	0	0
Blue Agave Nectar, Wholesome®, Organic, syrup, low glycemic	1 tsp	60	0	0	0
Equal®, packet	1 gram	0	0	0	0
Splenda®, packet	1 gram	0	0	0	0
Stevia Plus, Sweet Leaf®	¼ tsp	0	0	0	0
Sweet & Low®, packet	1 gram	0	0	0	0
Xylitol, Kal®	1 tsp	10	0	0	0

Chol (mg)	Sod (mg)	Carb (g)	Fiber (g)	Sugar (g)	Prot (g)
0	0	10	0	10	0
0	0	13	0	12 HF	0
0	0	13	0	12 HF	0
0	0	5	0	0 A	0
0	10	13	0	13 HF	0
0	10	13	0	13 HF	0

0	0	4	0	4	0
0	0	4	0	4	0
0	0	4	0	4	0
0	0	30	0	29	0
0	0	37	0	34	0
0	0	4	0	4	0
0	0	4	0	4	0
0	0	4	0	4	0
0	0	3	0	3	0
0	4	4	0	4	0
0	na	16	0	16	0
0	0	1	0	1 A	0
0	0	1	0	1 A	0
0	0	0	0	0	0
0	0	1	0	1 A	0
0	0	4	0	0	0

Discretionary or Optional Choices

Item	Serving	Cal	Total Fat (g)	Sat Fat (g)	Trans Fat (g)

SYRUP

Chocolate

Item	Serving	Cal	Total Fat (g)	Sat Fat (g)	Trans Fat (g)
AH!laska®, Organic	2 tbsp	100	0	0	0
Hershey's®	2 tbsp	100	0	0	0
Nestle®	2 tbsp	100	0	0	0

Corn

Item	Serving	Cal	Total Fat (g)	Sat Fat (g)	Trans Fat (g)
Brown Sugar, Karo®	2 tbsp	120	0	0	0
Dark	1 tbsp	57	0	0	0
High Fructose	1 tbsp	53	0	0	0
Light	1 tbsp	31	0	0	0
Vanilla, Wholesome®, Organic	½ cup	120	0	0	0
Vanilla, Karo®, lite	2 tbsp	120	0	0	0
Honey	1 tbsp	64	0	0	0
Molasses	1 tbsp	58	0	0	0

Pancake

Item	Serving	Cal	Total Fat (g)	Sat Fat (g)	Trans Fat (g)
Aunt Jemima®, original	¼ cup	210	0	0	0
Aunt Jemima®, light	¼ cup	100	0	0	0
Aunt Jemima®, Country Rich	¼ cup	210	0	0	0
Aunt Jemima®, Country Rich, light	¼ cup	100	0	0	0
Kellogg's, Eggo™, original	¼ cup	240	0	0	0
Kellogg's Eggo™, light	¼ cup	110	0	0	0
Log Cabin®, original	¼ cup	210	0	0	0
Log Cabin®, sugar free	¼ cup	35	0	0	0
Maple Grove Farms®, Pure Maple Syrup, Dark Amber, Organic	¼ cup	200	0	0	0
Maple Grove Farms®, sugar free	¼ cup	30	0	0	0
Mrs. Butterworth®, original	¼ cup	220	0	0	0
Mrs. Butterworth®, light	¼ cup	114	0	0	0
Naturally Preferred®, Maple Syrup, Organic	¼ cup	210	0	0	0
Santini®, Apricot, Syrup Organic	4 tbsp	214	0	0	0

Chol (mg)	Sod (mg)	Carb (g)	Fiber (g)	Sugar (g)	Prot (g)
0	0	25	0	22	1
0	0	25	0	20 HF	1
0	55	25	1	23	0
0	30	29	0	10	0
0	31	16	0	5	0
0	0	14	0	5	0
0	7	8	0	3	0
0	30	30	0	30	0
0	35	31	0	12 HF	0
0	1	17	0	17	0
0	7	15	0	11	0
0	120	52	0	32 HF	0
0	190	26	1	25 HF	0
0	120	53	0	30 HF	0
0	180	26	1	25 HF	0
0	35	↑60	0	40 HF	0
0	180	27	0	25 HF	0
0	100	53	0	39 HF	0
0	100	12	0	0 A	0
0	5	53	0	53	0
0	110	11	0	0 A	0
0	130	55	0	38 HF	0
0	130	25	0	24 HF	0
0	5	53	0	53	0
0	112	51	0	51	2

Discretionary or Optional Choices

Item	Serving	Cal	Total Fat (g)	Sat Fat (g)	Trans Fat (g)
Pancake, Syrup *continued*					
Santini®, Blueberry, Organic	4 tbsp	214	0	0	0
Santini®, Honey Pecan, Organic	4 tbsp	214	0	0	0
Santini®, Maple, Organic	4 tbsp	214	0	0	0
Rice Syrup, Lundberg®, Organic, Brown Rice Syrup	2 tbsp	150	0	0	0

Chol (mg)	Sod (mg)	Carb (g)	Fiber (g)	Sugar (g)	Prot (g)
0	112	51	0	51	2
0	112	51	0	51	2
0	112	51	0	51	2
0	70	35	0	22	0

Soups

Soups can be a side dish, hearty meal or used as a flavorful sauce for meats, poultry, seafood or vegetables. Soups can fall into one or more of the USDA Pyramid Food Groups, i.e. the Vegetable Group, Grain Group and/or the Meat and Bean Group.

Soups are packed with vitamins and minerals from a variety of food groups.

Soups made with vegetables, beans and lentils are ↑ **in fiber.**

Soups with meat, poultry or seafood contain **cholesterol** and may be ↑ **higher in fat** than vegetable or broth based soups.

Dry soup mixes, bouillon cubes or powders may contain **Trans Fats** (partially hydrogenated oils). Products containing Partially Hydrogenated Oils are coded with a [P] in this chapter.

Many soups contain 20% and up to 50% of the recommended Daily Value for **sodium** based on a 2,000 calorie diet. Most soups are ↑ **in sodium** even low sodium varieties.

Compare "Chicken Broths" in this chapter. Find the brand with the least amount of sodium. If you chose the brand with 130mg, you've just saved yourself anywhere from 440mg to 1140mg of sodium. And guess what—zero Trans Fats (no partially hydrogenated oils)!

EAT SMART. Compare brands to reduce sodium. Select soups ↑ in fiber more often. Check the INGREDIENTS list for "partially hydrogenated" oils and avoid Trans Fat.

Item	Serving	Cal	Total Fat (g)	Sat Fat (g)	Trans Fat (g)
SOUPS					
Beef					
Campbell's®, Beef Broth	1 cup	15	0	0	0
Campbell's®, Vegetable Beef	1 cup	90	1	.5	0
Campbell's® Select, Beef with Roasted Barley	1 cup	130	1	.5	0
Progresso® Traditional, Beef & Mushroom	1 cup	100	.5	0	0
Progresso®, Traditional, Beef & Vegetable	1 cup	100	1	0	0
Top Ramen®, Nissin®, beef flavor, dry, prepared	½ pkg	190	7	↑3.5	0
Beef Broth					
Swanson's®, canned	1 cup	15	0	0	0
Swanson's®, 33% less sodium, canned	1 cup	15	0	0	0
Wyler®, Bouillon Cube, prepared	1 cup	0	0	0	0 ᴾ
Black Bean					
Amy's®, Black Bean Vegetable	1 cup	130	1.5	0	0
Campbell's®, Black Bean	1 cup	110	1.5	.5	0
Muir Glen®, Southwest Black Bean, Organic	1 cup	130	1	0	0
Butternut Squash					
Amy's®, Organic, low fat	1 cup	100	2.5	0	0
Amy's®, Organic, light sodium	1 cup	100	2.5	0	0
Pacific Natural®, Organic, carton	1 cup	90	2	0	0
Pacific Natural®, Organic, light sodium, carton	1 cup	90	2	0	0
Chicken					
Campbell's®, Chicken Noodle	1 cup	60	2	.5	0
Campbell's®, Chicken Noodle, 25% less sodium	1 cup	60	2	.5	0
Campbell's®, Chicken Noodle, dry mix, prepared	1 cup	100	1.5	.5	0 ᴾ

Chol (mg)	Sod (mg)	Carb (g)	Fiber (g)	Sugar (g)	Prot (g)
0	⬆860	1	0	1	3
5	⬆890	15	3	2	5
10	⬆920	22	2	4	9
15	⬆960	13	1	3	7
15	⬆850	17	2	4	7
0	⬆760	27	2	0	5
0	⬆890	1	0	0	2
0	440	1	0	0	3
0	⬆990	0	0	0	0
0	430	25	⬆5	6	6
0	⬆960	18	⬆6	5	6
0	⬆680	25	⬆8	4	7
0	⬆580	20	2	4	2
0	290	20	2	4	2
0	⬆550	17	3	4	2
0	280	17	3	4	2
15	⬆890	8	1	1	6
15	⬆660	8	1	1	3
20	⬆810	17	1	2	4

Discretionary or Optional Choices

Item	Serving	Cal	Total Fat (g)	Sat Fat (g)	Trans Fat (g)
Chicken, Soup *continued*					
Campbell's®, Cream of Chicken, 98% fat free	1 cup	70	2.5	1	0
Progresso®, Traditional, Chicken Noodle	1 cup	100	2.5	.5	0
Progresso®, Chicken Noodle, low sodium	1 cup	90	1.5	0	0
Top Ramen®, Nissin®, chicken flavor, dry, prepared	½ pkg	190	7	⬆3.5	0
Chicken Broth					
Campbell's®, Broth	1 cup	20	1	0	0
Health Valley®, Organic, Broth	1 cup	35	1.5	.5	0
Knorr®, Bouillon Cubes, prepared	1 cup	20	1.5	.5	0 ᴾ
Swanson®, Broth	1 cup	10	.5	0	0
Swanson®, Broth, 33% less sodium	1 cup	15	0	0	0
Wyler®, Bouillon Cubes, prepared	1 cup	5	0	0	0 ᴾ
Corn Chowder					
Amy's®	1 cup	190	10	⬆4.5	0
Progresso®, Rich & Hearty	1 cup	210	9	2.5	0
Clam Chowder					
Campbell's®, New England	1 cup	90	2.5	.5	0
Campbell's® Select, New England, 98% fat free	1 cup	110	1.5	0	0
Chunky™, Campbell's®, New England Clam Chowder	1 cup	190	9	2	0
Progresso®, Rich & Hearty, New England Clam Chowder	1 cup	190	9	2	0
Onion					
Campbell's® French Onion	1 cup	45	1.5	1	0
Lipton®, Beefy Onion, dry mix, prepared	1 cup	25	.5	0	0 ᴾ

Chol (mg)	Sod (mg)	Carb (g)	Fiber (g)	Sugar (g)	Prot (g)
10	↑590	10	1	1	1
25	↑950	12	1	1	7
20	↑470	12	1	2	7
0	↑910	26	2	1	5
5	↑770	1	0	1	1
0	130	0	0	0	5
0	↑1270	1	0	1	1
5	↑960	1	0	1	1
0	↑570	1	0	1	3
0	↑880	1	0	0	0
25	↑580	25	3	4	3
15	↑790	23	2	5	7
5	↑880	13	1	1	4
10	↑850	18	2	2	5
10	↑890	21	2	2	6
10	↑840	22	2	2	6
5	↑900	6	1	4	2
0	↑590	5	1	0	0

Discretionary or Optional Choices

Item	Serving	Cal	Total Fat (g)	Sat Fat (g)	Trans Fat (g)
Onion, Soup *continued*					
Lipton®, Onion Soup, dry mix, prepared	1 cup	20	0	0	0 ᴾ
Pacific Natural®, French Onion, Organic	1 cup	35	0	0	0
Progresso® Vegetable Classic, French Onion	1 cup	50	1.5	.5	0
Lentil					
Campbell's®, Savory Lentil	1 cup	140	.5	.5	0
Muir Glen®, Savory Lentil, Organic	1 cup	130	2	1	0
Pacific Natural®, Curried Red Lentil	1 cup	140	4.5	↑4	0
Progresso® Vegetable Classic, Lentil	1 cup	150	2	.5	0
Minestrone					
Amy's®, Organic, low fat	1 cup	90	1.5	0	0
Amy's®, Organic, light sodium	1 cup	90	1.5	0	0
Campbell's®, Minestrone	1 cup	90	1	.5	0
Health Valley®, Minestrone, Organic	1 cup	100	2	0	0
Muir Glen®, Classic Minestrone, Organic	1 cup	110	2	1	0
Progresso® Traditional, Minestrone with Chicken	1 cup	120	3.5	.5	0
Progresso® Vegetable Classic, 99% fat free	1 cup	100	1	0	0
Progresso®, 50% less sodium	1 cup	120	2	.5	0
Pea					
Amy's®, Split Pea, Organic, fat free	1 cup	100	0	0	0
Campbell's®, Green Pea	1 cup	180	3	1	0
Muir Glen®, Home Style Split Pea, Organic	1 cup	170	1	0	0
Tomato					
Amy's®, Chunky Tomato Bisque	1 cup	120	3.5	2	0
Amy's®, Chunky Tomato Bisque, light sodium	1 cup	120	3.5	2	0
Campbell's®, Tomato	1 cup	90	0	0	0

Chol (mg)	Sod (mg)	Carb (g)	Fiber (g)	Sugar (g)	Prot (g)
0	↑610	4	1	0	0
0	↑660	6	1	2	1
5	↑850	8	1	3	1
0	↑790	27	↑6	5	8
0	↑900	35	↑5	4	10
0	↑750	19	↑5	8	5
0	↑870	28	↑5	1	9
0	↑580	19	3	5	3
0	280	19	3	5	3
5	↑960	17	3	3	4
0	70	17	3	5	4
0	↑960	19	↑5	3	4
15	↑870	16	3	2	6
0	↑630	19	4	3	5
0	↑470	24	4	4	5
0	↑670	19	3	4	7
0	↑870	28	4	6	9
0	↑900	35	↑5	4	10
10	↑680	21	2	0	14
10	340	21	2	0	14
0	↑770	20	1	12	2

Discretionary or Optional Choices

Item	Serving	Cal	Total Fat (g)	Sat Fat (g)	Trans Fat (g)
Tomato, Soup *continued*					
Campbell's®, Tomato, 25% less sodium	1 cup	90	0	0	0
Muir Glen®, Creamy Tomato, Organic	1 cup	170	6	2	0
Muir Glen®, Hearty Tomato, Organic	1 cup	130	2	1	0
Pacific Natural®, Organic	1 cup	100	2	1.5	.5
Pacific Natural®, Organic, light sodium	1 cup	100	2	1.5	.5
Progresso®, Hearty Tomato	1 cup	110	1	0	0
Vegetable					
Amy's®, Chunky Vegetable, fat free	1 cup	60	0	0	0
Campbell's®, Vegetable	1 cup	100	.5	.5	0
Muir Glen®, Garden Vegetable, Organic	1 cup	80	1	0	0
Progresso®, Garden Vegetable, low sodium	1 cup	100	0	0	0

Chol (mg)	Sod (mg)	Carb (g)	Fiber (g)	Sugar (g)	Prot (g)
0	↑530	20	1	12	2
15	↑840	26	2	16	4
0	↑880	25	2	19	5
10	↑750	16	1	12	5
10	380	16	1	12	5
0	↑980	23	3	9	2
0	↑680	13	3	5	3
5	↑890	20	3	7	4
0	↑960	16	3	5	3
0	450	22	3	4	3

Codes and Abbreviations

Cal = calories
Carb = carbohydrates
Chol = cholesterol
Prot = protein
Sat fat = saturated fat
Sod = sodium
Serv = serving

g = gram
med = medium
mg = milligrams
na = not available
oz = ounce
pkg = package
pkt = packet
sm = small
tbsp = tablespoon
tsp = teaspoon
w/ = with
w/o = without

Complete = "just add water" a term used for many packaged (dry) mixes.

Dry = not cooked or prepared.

Prep or prepared = prepared according to directions. Items such as meat, butter, oil, etc., added during preparation are calculated into the Nutrition Facts.

Unprepared = not prepared. Items such as meat, butter, oil, etc., added during preparation are not calculated into the Nutrition Facts.

^{A} = Artificial Sweetener

^{P} = Partially Hydrogenated Oil

^{H} = Hydrogenated Fat

^{E} = Enriched Grains

^{HF} = High Fructose Corn Syrup

^{W} = Whole Grains

^{R} = Refined Grains

↑ = High (20% or more) in this nutrient

References

USDA National Nutrient Database for Standard Reference, Release 19; NUTRITION FACT labels; Product INGREDIENT lists.

Daily Servings and Daily Values, Center for Food Safety and Applied Nutrition (CFSAN); www.mypyramid.gov; United Stated Department of Agriculture (USDA); Millions of Americans don't understand nutrition (approximately 95% of Americans don't understand nutrition and dietary terms, the American Journal of Clinical Nutrition).

Artificial Sweeteners—Ruth Kava, PhD, RD, Director of nutrition for the American Council on Science and Health, Are Artificial Sweeteners Safe?; Paula Baillie-Hamilton, M.D., PhD, author of *Toxic Overload*; Sharon P. Fowler, MPH, University of Texas Health Science Center, American Diabetes Association 65th Annual meeting, 2005; Harvard Medical School Artificial Sweeteners and Health; Food and Drug Administration, Acceptable Daily Intake; Sweetleaf® Stevia; Blue Agave Nectar®; The University of Sydney www.glycemicindex.com.

High Fructose Corn Syrup—University of Cincinnati research study on fructose and body fat; Dr. Mehmet Oz, Red Flag Ingredients; WebMD HFCS Linked to Extra Calories; American Journal of Clinical Nutrition, Consumption of HFCS in Beverages, George A. Bray, Samara Joy Neilson and Barry M. Popkin.

Hydrogenated Fat—USDA, What are Solid Fats; Food and Nutrition Center (FNIC) Nutrition Information Specialist, email response April 20th, 2007.

Partially Hydrogenated Oils—University of Maryland, Trans Fats 101; Food and Drug Administration; Good Fats Bad Fats, Rosemary Stanton, Ph.D.; Trans Fat Translation, Robert L. Wolke, Professor emeritus of chemistry University of Pittsburgh.

What Are Carbohydrates—Whole Grain Foods and Risk of Heart Disease and Certain Cancers Docket No. 99P-2209; CFSAN/FDA, Fiber-Containing Grain Products, Fruits, and Vegetables and Cancer – 21 CFR 101.76; Fruits, Vegetables and Grain Products that contain Fiber, particularly Soluble Fiber, and Risk of Coronary Heart Disease – 21 CFR 101.77.

Nuts and Seeds—American Diabetes Association, In A Nutshell; Harvard University, Nuts and Your Health;

Cracking Old Myths, Center for Food Safety and Applied Nutrition; FDA, Qualified Health Claims; Nuts and Coronary Heart Disease Docket No. 02P-0505; Mayo Clinic, How Fish Helps Your Heart (Omega-3); American Heart Association, Journal Report, – Almonds have cholesterol benefits; USDA National Nutrient Database for Standard Reference – Release 19.

Beef, Pork and Lamb—USDA/Agriculture Marketing Services, How to buy meat; Medline plus Cholesterol; Jeanne Goldberg PHD., 50 ways to lower your fat and cholesterol; Nutrition Labeling and Education Act of 1990 (NLEA); www.mypyramid.gov; American Cancer Society, controlling portions; Food Safety and Information services, Meat and Poultry Labeling Terms; Survey: Restaurants dishing out extra-large portions by Nanci Hellmich, USA Today; Center for Food Safety and Applied Nutrition, The Label Dictionary; Meat information extracted from the USDA National Nutrient Database for Standard Reference, Release 19 is based on "all grades" of cooked meat unless otherwise noted, separable lean and fat trimmed to 1/4" to 1/8".

Fish and Shellfish—FDA/EPA Advisory on Seafood Consumption/FDA Statement June 6, 2006; Mayo Clinic, Fish FAQ The Merits and hazards of eating fish; Environmental Working Group's Fish list—high level data obtained from FDA documents; Dr. Perricone, *The Wrinkle Free Diet*; American Heart Association; American Diabetes Association; American Cancer Society; FDA/EPA Advisory on Seafood Consumption, June 6, 2006.

The Milk Group—Mid West Dairy Association; Shamrock Foods; USDA, How to Buy Cheese.

Oils—Spectrum oils www.spectrumorganics.com; North Dakota State University; Sunflowers – Oleic and Linoleic, National Sunflower Association.

Dairy and Non Dairy—Center for food safety and Applied Nutrition (CFSAN): A Food Labeling Guide.

Herbs, Spices, Salt—Salt Works Inc. www.seasalt.com; American Heart Association; Health Dilemmas—Has Salt gotten a bad Shake, www.TheVegetarianTimes.com ; USDA recommended Daily Values for Sodium.

Jelly, Jams, Sweeteners and Syrup—Smucker's Company; www.dickensonsfamily.com; Cascadian Farms.

Creating Balance
Seminars & Consulting Services

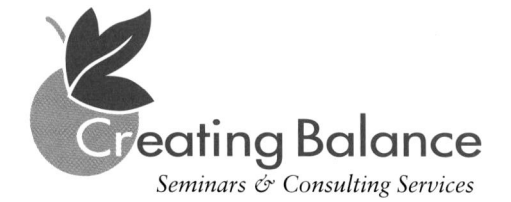

For more information about Seminars and Consulting Services contact Celeste Bumpus:

Phone: 602-430-2786
Email: celeste@creatingbalanceseminars.com
Online: www.cr-eatingbalance.com
Mail: 21001 N. Tatum Blvd.
Ste. 1630-458
Phoenix, Arizona 85050

Thank You!

About the Author

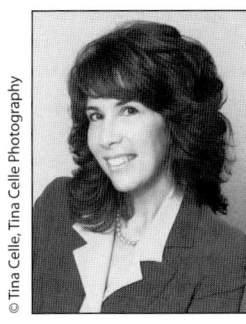

Celeste Bumpus is a professional speaker, consultant and president of Creating Balance Seminars.

A former General Manager for American Express Corporate Services, Celeste worked her way up from an entry-level position to managing over 25 business locations.

As a mother of two, Celeste understands the challenges many people face with juggling a career, family and/or maintaining a healthy lifestyle.

A savvy shopper and product expert, Celeste reviews hundreds of whole and processed foods each year. "Processed foods are a reality in today's world. As with any type food, there are good and not so good choices."

Knowledge and organizational skills were keys to her mastering a healthy work/life balance. Recognizing that eating healthy is a skill and simple changes can add up, Celeste formed Creating Balance Seminars to help others achieve a healthier lifestyle.

From bottom lines to waistlines, business planning to meal planning, Celeste partners with companies and associations who want to create a healthier environment for leaders and employees. Celeste delivers fundamental life-changing information "in plain English" empowering individuals to eat smart and take charge of their lives.

"What I've found is most people want to eat healthy and maintain a healthy lifestyle, but they're either too busy or they don't know how. My goal is to make eating healthy easier."

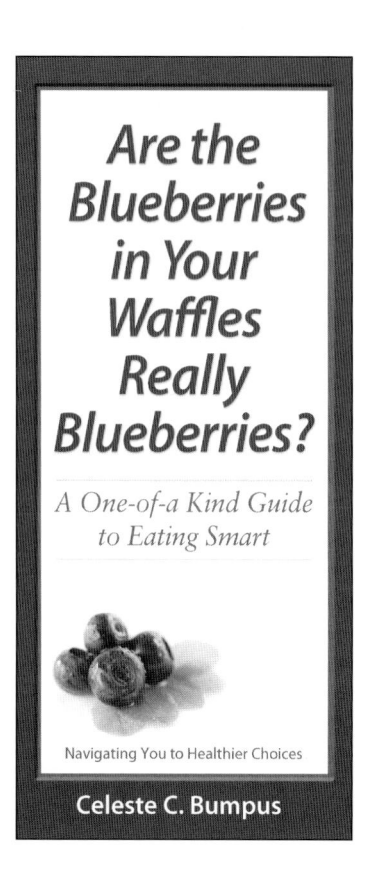

> ## *Are the Blueberries in Your Waffles Really Blueberries?*
>
> *A One-of-a Kind Guide to Eating Smart*
>
> Navigating You to Healthier Choices
>
> **Celeste C. Bumpus**

Are the Blueberries in Your Waffles Really Blueberries?

A One-of-a Kind Guide to Eating Smart

ISBN-13: 978-0-9790820-0-9 / U.S. $19.99

To find out about volume discounts on orders of 10 or more copies for individuals, corporations, associations or as gifts, please contact us at 602-430-2786 or via email at eatsmart@cr-eatingbalance.com